"*On the Sweet Spot* is a great book. It is much more than just a 'how to improve at golf psychology' book. Fun reading and insightful, you won't want to put this book down."

—Hank Haney, legendary golf instructor

"Richard Keefe was extremely helpful to me as I prepared mentally for the Masters and the PGA Tour. Many of his best lessons are in this brilliant book, *On the Sweet Spot*. It is sure to help golfers play their best and enjoy themselves more."

—Tim Clark, PGA Tour, four-time NCAA All-America

"*On the Sweet Spot* is a gift to every golfer, regardless of skill level, who chases the elusive dream of consistently playing their best golf. By pursuing 'the effortless present,' we quiet the mind that can derail our swings, and we enrich our lives and spirits. In sharing his journey, Dr. Keefe has shortened the road we all travel."

—Ed Ibarguen, Top-100 Teacher, *Golf Magazine*; General Manager and PGA Director of Golf, Duke University Golf Club

"*On the Sweet Spot* is a stimulating book dedicated to helping everyone understand their performance potential. I found the neuropsychological implications fascinating! Dr. Keefe has done a wonderful job of providing a story and the psychological insight needed to help athletes and coaches achieve athletic genius!"

—Robert K. Winters, Ph.D., Resident Sport Psychologist, David Leadbetter Golf Academy

"Richard Keefe has crafted a brilliant work, certain to become a bible for golfers and other athletes. His message is far broader, however, encouraging the pursuit of sport, work, and love as spiritual art forms. Dr. Keefe masterfully weaves diverse threads from sport psychology, modern cognitive neuroscience, philosophy, and theology into a rich tapestry that lets viewers enjoy its warmth. The brain science is solid and rendered with lucidity, easy accessibility for the nonscientist, and humor all too rare among researchers. Rich in both instruction and poignancy, *On the Sweet Spot* is an essential read for everyone who thinks about how they are moved, be it in their sport or in their lives."

—Robert M. Bilder, Ph.D., ABPP, Professor of Psychiatry and Biobehavioral Sciences, Chief of Medical Psychology–Neuropsychology, Brain Mapping Center, UCLA

"*On The Sweet Spot* weaves mountains of practical sport psychology into a fascinating story line that is sure to help athletes at every level."

—Jay Lapidus, Duke University Men's Tennis Coach

"Dr. Keefe, in *On the Sweet Spot*, provides a unique and engaging view of the paths that people take to optimal athletic performance. In doing so, he highlights the importance of that seemingly effortless state where remarkable athletic achievement often occurs. He also breaks down the processes governing these near-mystical states into clear steps. Dr. Keefe maps these steps onto brain circuits and builds from these insights to consider both performance problems and performance-enhancing strategies. Dr. Keefe succeeds in linking opposing perspectives on performance (subjective and objective, religious and scientific, instinctive and strategic) because he draws on his own experience as an athlete, a clinical psychologist, and a leading cognitive neuroscientist. Perhaps, not surprisingly, the lessons learned about athletic achievement in this book have important implications for success in other areas of one's life."

—**John H. Krystal, M.D., Albert E. Kent Professor and Deputy Chairman for Research, Department of Psychiatry, Yale University School of Medicine**

"Belief in one's self is by far the most important skill a golfer must develop; in my view, 'staying in the present' is all about belief. *On the Sweet Spot* provides scientific support for the crucial role such belief plays in elite performance—and in living a full life. This book's optimistic message provides hope for us all: What we need to be better people, to be better performers, is in us already. Dr. Keefe has tapped into the physiological and evolutionary underpinnings of the most fascinating aspects of being human."

—**Dan Brooks, Head Coach, Duke Women's Golf, 2002 NCAA Champions**

"*On the Sweet Spot* is a wonderfully practical book. It helps readers understand the connection between brain function, psychology, and peak performance. Readers interested in enhancing their athletic performance or their life performance will find helpful ideas to put into practice today. All of us have had brief moments in 'the zone' athletically or otherwise, and all of us want to go back there. This book shows you how."

—**Dr. Daniel Amen, author of *Change Your Brain, Change Your Life* and *Healing the Hardware of the Soul***

"If you've ever thought that golf is a mental game, you absolutely have to read this book. In my thirty years of working on the mental side of golf, I've consulted for dozens of PGA Tour players who at times have played golf in a way that was somehow special yet effortless. In *On the Sweet Spot*, Dr. Keefe eloquently describes the mental state behind this kind of performance, and provides tremendously useful input about how every player can achieve it on and off the course."

—**Dr. Richard Coop, author of *Mind Over Golf*, and special consultant to *Golf Magazine***

"Richard Keefe has written a book that will help you improve your performance in any area of your life, from driving to work to pondering the mind of God."

—**Redford Williams, M.D., author of *Anger Kills***

On the Sweet Spot

STALKING THE EFFORTLESS PRESENT

Dr. Richard Keefe

SIMON & SCHUSTER

NEW YORK   LONDON   TORONTO   SYDNEY   SINGAPORE

SIMON & SCHUSTER
Rockefeller Center
1230 Avenue of the Americas
New York, NY 10020

For information regarding special discounts for bulk purchases,
please contact Simon & Schuster Special Sales:
1-800-456-6798 or business@simonandschuster.com

Manufactured in the United States of America

3   5   7   9   10   8   6   4

Library of Congress Cataloging-in-Publication Data
Keefe, Richard S. E.
On the sweet spot : stalking the effortless present / Richard Keefe
p.   cm.
Includes bibliographical references and index.
1. Golf—Psychological aspects.   I. Title.
GV979.P75 K43   2003
796.352'01'9—dc21   2002042778
ISBN-13: 978-1-5011-2585-0

For Caren and our children

CONTENTS

PROLOGUE

A BABY TWISTED uncomfortably in her mother's lap. She was only three weeks old, and had no idea what she was doing. Her belly hurt, but she didn't know that; the pain sensors in her stomach sent a signal to her brain, precipitating a message to move the area. This all happened instantaneously. She yelped in anguish, and thrust her midsection from side to side. Her mother saw her pain; patted her tiny, seemingly frail, back; then gently laid her into the crook of one arm to feed her. Even before the milk reached the baby's belly, her pain was erased by a feeling of satisfaction that was so powerful, so all-encompassing, that her body went limp and her cries were not even a memory. She felt a bliss that her mother and father could no longer know.

There were so many steps between her longing and her satisfaction, but she was aware of none of them. She knew the longing—its tumultuous crash into the depths of her being, leaving her tiny world in chaos. She also knew its cessation—the way her body and her spirit responded with peace when that longing was addressed. But the mechanism, her mother's love assuring that her longing led to satisfaction, was beyond her perception. It felt to her as though her needs were being met as if of their own accord: she longed, and was satisfied. Trillions of connections among the neurons in her brain shrunk and grew so that she could have this experi-

1

ence again and again. The connections formed at a furious pace, like the blooming of spring, creating neural pathways dependent upon the world she encountered. In this morning, in the half-dawn, she encountered the satisfaction of her longing; it overpowered her, and its presence soothed her. Though she was yet unable to feel her awe, her faith in the love that enveloped her grew steadily. And, as her faith and her neural connections grew, a door inside her opened to the direct experience of God.

CHAPTER ONE

Spontaneous Generation

I DID NOT REALLY TRUST the orthopedist who was about to operate on my knee. Maybe that was why I wanted to stay awake during the surgery. A friend of mine who was an M.D. told me it was safer not to have general anesthesia, and I was nervous about the surgery, even though it was minor. I don't really remember why I was afraid. Perhaps it was because I was thirty-two at the time, and my life felt so empty. I had just finished graduate school in clinical psychology a year before, and was having trouble finding much inspiration in my new position as a faculty member in a psychiatry department. Each day of research on the causes of schizophrenia seemed to be fraught with interpersonal battles disguised as politics disguised as scientific inquiry. My personal life had no future either: I was dating a young woman who had just finished college and lived with her mother. I was on the cusp of middle age, and she was dyeing her hair a new color each month and wondering what it would be like to have a job. I guess being with her helped me ignore the fact that time was racing along, and I was stuck by the side of the road with a flat tire. What if I were to die or become crippled during the operation? Who would be there to care about what had happened? Who would know about all the plans I had made?

Lying flat on my back in the operating room, with nothing but a flimsy hospital gown-thing draped over me, I discussed with the anesthesiologist my preference to stay awake during the surgery; she seemed a little chagrined, but accepting. The orthopedist would have none of it: I recall him storming into the operating room, not even breaking stride as he said, "That's okay if you don't want a general anesthetic," getting me to open up in optimistic anticipation, "but I won't be doing the surgery." Punch in the stomach. Now, I had done a bad thing. Of course I would relinquish my tiny little toy gun in the presence of someone holding a nuclear weapon. I had angered a man about to pierce my flesh while I was unconscious. I don't remember what I said next; I only remember someone fitting a gas mask onto my face and counting backward from ten.

When I awoke, my red-haired girlfriend (wasn't she blonde when I went under?) and a friend of mine who was a psychiatrist at the hospital were there. I had hoped that having nearby a friend who was on the medical staff at the hospital would somehow get me better treatment, or even save my life if it were endangered. But my orthopedist, who obviously preferred to have people unconscious, had little respect for my psychiatrist buddy, whose job it was to make people less unconscious. As it turned out, though, I needed someone with a caring demeanor to break the news to me: The orthopedist had enlisted my friend to explain to me that my years of playing sports had completely worn down my knee, and that the little pain I was having was the burning friction of bone against bone. I would never again be able to participate in vigorous athletic activity.

I was devastated initially, but this feeling strangely lifted after about an hour. When I had recovered enough from the surgery to be discharged, and the anesthesia diminished to a pleasant afterglow, my girlfriend drove me home in my convertible. We stopped along the way for her to go to a hair appointment, and I waited in the car, pondering my loss of identity as an athlete so intently that I didn't even notice that when she got back in the car she was a brunette.

We drove along through the older, richer, back roads of Westchester County, and passed a vast expanse of fields and trees, encircled by a century-old, waist-high stone wall. The April afternoon was warm and cloudy, pregnant with new life and the possibility of rain. On the other side of the stone wall, small groups of people were hovering near each other, moving in clumps along the field. My cognitive functions had been slowed by the pain medication and, for about a full minute, I did not know what they were doing. I felt a longing to be with them, engaged in their activity, but I had no idea what it was. The emotional centers of my brain were unaffected by the lingering effects of the medication, but my analytical abilities were shut down. I did not dwell considerably upon what I didn't know about their activity; rather, I bathed in my longing. I felt a primal need to be with these people, doing whatever it was that they were doing. I did not even know if they were working or playing. It seemed to be both. Farther up the road, the sight of a woman pulling a flagstick out of the ground broke my state of cerebral numbness. Golf. They were playing *golf*.

I immediately became excited at the prospect of it. Perhaps this would pull me out of my little identity crisis. I would still be able to walk, and I could probably swing a club without hurting my knee, although I'd have to test this when I was healthy again. Yes, I was excited about this. The embarrassingly intense longing that I'd felt could, in fact, be satisfied. When I was a teenager I had had a period of playing golf every day for a single summer. At the time, I'd quit because I began to feel like I was playing an old man's game, and was pulled into the local orbit of my buddies playing team sports. Now, ironically, I associated golf with youth, and didn't even think about how the swift insertion of an arthroscope into my knee had sentenced my body to middle age as quickly as Dr. Knock-you-out could say "sedated." Golf meant endless adolescent summer days to me: Warm up by putting on your shoes, then play forty-five; go home for dinner, come back the next day. Only in retrospect can I see the human resiliency in my sudden revitalization. Part of it may have been a quirk in the timing of my brain's recovery from the pain medication: I could recall my intense, youthful joy without quite knowing what was making me happy. I felt as though a course had been set: I would play golf. My knee would not hinder me there. I was young again.

I found that my knee injury did not affect my swing at all, and the walking was therapeutic. I started off slowly at first, hitting balls occasionally, practicing my putting, then playing six-hour rounds when I was able to get onto the crowded New York area courses. Several months later, after haircolor girl had told me on Thanksgiving night that she was seeing a younger man—*while we were in the bathtub together*—I met my future wife. She was friends with a group of tennis players who also played golf, and I began to play and practice with increasing frequency. The depth of my relationship with this woman, and with the game that would infuse my life, grew in parallel. One of her friends, as well as her parents, lived in Suffern, New York, which permits residents to play at Spook Rock Golf Club, one of the finest municipal courses in the United States. Since she never had the patience for golf, she would socialize with our group on the practice range, then visit her parents while I played. As I warmed up on the range, my focus on golf would begin to narrow, and my attention to her and the others would become fleeting, almost false. As our foursome packed up to head for the first tee, she would kiss me goodbye and say, "have fun," but I had already left. It was as though we were now characters in two completely different movies. She was in a romantic comedy, making jokes with her husband and their friends, immersed in the interaction of the people around her. I was in a war epic; my kiss goodbye was dramatic, perhaps final, as I headed off into an unknown land of potential heroics and unspeakable lurking horrors. My return was much the same: I had battles to speak of, some of them bloody. She asked incomprehensible questions, such as, "Did you have a nice time?" The contrast in our communication was like a dream, where bizarre and incongruous events are treated with nonchalance.

    I: That two-tongued half-lizard, half-man is going to kill us!
She: Tea?

As my interest in golf flourished, I looked for any opportunity to play or practice. I developed a real love of hitting balls. I would practice for hours, standing behind the ball, picturing the exact flight that the ball would take, the exact swing that I would make. Then, I would approach the ball, get into my stance, and try to make the image I had created transform itself through me into a golf shot. When I was successful, I felt a great inner satisfaction. I felt as though I had a special gift, that I was able to enter into a mental state where I could turn my inner pictures into real events in the outer world. It was this extraordinary feeling, more than any other, that drove me. I felt, in each swing, that I was creating a work of art. I was making an internal image come to life. The process made me feel powerful and confident. I recalled the time in my youth when I had rejected golf, feeling that it was a meaningless activity; quite the contrary now, I felt there was something elemental in what I was doing. I felt such a basic intensity that I could have been running through the jungle, chasing my prey fifty thousand years ago, or confidently making a complicated, delicate maneuver to dock a spaceship to a space station, far in the future.

This intensity brought a tremendous joy to my life. I practiced in the evenings, played on the weekends, and spent the rest of my free time with my wife-to-be. The progress of research into the causes of mental illnesses moves slowly, and uninspired researchers like me at the time can easily get lost in the meandering crowd if they wish. I had plenty of free time if I wanted it; I didn't miss any important meetings, but I missed the unimportant ones. In a research career, there are nine bad ideas being pursued for every good one. I simply cut loose a few of the projects that were going nowhere. I sometimes worry that, by doing so, I cut loose the cure for mental illness. This is unlikely; when I looked around my department, I saw a number of people who were wasting a lot more than a few ideas. I again felt as though time were racing along, but I was no longer an observer; some of the others now seemed stuck by the side of the road, while I was flowing with the traffic in the open air. The breeze was light and the sun was warm. I felt my hands as they grasped the wheel.

When my wife-to-be and I became engaged to be married, I moved from Westchester County, New York, to Bergen County, New Jersey. This move tore me away from a region steeped in some of golf's greatest history and tradition, to an area that was ranked as the third-worst county in the United States for golf. There were four county courses, and each one was terrible. I played them whenever I could. After all, the closest I've ever gotten to the Westchester courses like Winged Foot was watching Davis Love III win the PGA championship on television. Furthermore, a mile from our apartment in Edgewater was a driving range with a putting green. It was located on a converted landfill along the Hudson River, in the heart of a Korean section of the county, and the owners of the range were Korean, as well. It had the only snack room at a golf practice facility I have ever seen that sold a variety of green teas. Some evenings, with the 100 or so stalls two-deep in people waiting to pound jumbo buckets of 200-plus balls, I was the only non-Asian there.

I took comfort in the company of my equally obsessed brothers-in-arms. I sometimes practiced deep into the evening, as the lighted range was open until midnight (a happy fact that prompted a lawsuit by the tenants of the Manhattan apartment buildings across the Hudson, who were kept awake by the glaring lights). During the winter, the range was heated, and each stall was encased on three sides by thick, insulating plastic. During a strange weather period that included a series of ice storms, the range was covered in a thick blanket of ice, and each shot skittered and bounced along as though frictionless, until it found the net at the back of the range. This was the first time that I had been able to work on my swing through a winter, and the dramatic improvements made me wonder how professional golfers could ever be raised outside of southern climes.

At times, when I practiced, I had a vague feeling of a presence with me. It was sometimes the inner chattering of my mind, perhaps half words and part phrases directed toward improving my swing: *Hands there . . . loose, uh-huh . . . through to finish, like that . . . felt the big muscles that time . . . yuh.* When the chattering died down and my focus improved, the presence remained, hanging there. One day, quite suddenly, a warm and pleasing sensation spread through my chest. I felt happy and sad at the same time, and I felt vulnerable, yet safe. I was somewhat confused by all this, and was reminded of the time when I had first fallen in love with my wife. As I stood pondering all these different feelings, I developed a distinct and startling impression that I was not alone.

A few weeks later, as I practiced at the range in the summer, I again had the feeling of a presence with me. At first, it was like background music—a nice accompaniment that seemed to comfort me as I hit each shot. It then became fuller and more encompassing. My swing felt particularly fluid that day, and I was amazed at my ability to visualize the exact trajectory of where I wanted the ball to go, and then to manifest that same image by hitting the ball just right. I worked on moving the ball from left to right and right to left around the different flags that covered the practice area, and never felt more in control of making the ball go wherever I wanted it to. Yet, I had a strange feeling that it was not me swinging the club. It wasn't that I felt as though I were possessed, or taken over by an alien force, or anything weird like that. It was just that I felt I didn't need to put forth any effort to swing the club. The initial part of my swing, when I first brought the club back, was happening on its own. It seemed at times that the club was swinging itself. I had an impulse to head out onto the course and play a quick round, figuring that I shouldn't waste all these great shots on the practice range, but I was so enthralled and focused on what I was doing, I just kept hitting away.

I decided to experiment. I aimed at a telephone pole that held up the net at the back of the practice range, about 250 yards away. The ground was very hard and dry, so my best drives could hit the net after a few bounces. I got behind the ball and aligned myself toward the pole, then saw a picture of my drive sailing off toward the net, bouncing twice, and landing solidly against the pole. I even heard the distant *plonk* of the ball smacking against the wood, like a broom handle on a coconut. As I got into my stance and readied myself to swing, I completely let go of any feeling of *trying* to hit the shot. Years before, I had read a book about Zen Buddhist archers who draw back their bows then, rather than shoot the arrow, wait for the arrow to be loosed toward the target. I followed the same approach: I waited for the club to be swung. I did not try. I only waited. When the club finally began moving back, I felt almost as though I were an observer. I knew they were my hands, and my club, and my torso twisting my weight onto my right foot, but I felt that the swing was being started, and completed, as if of its own accord. Just as I had pictured seconds before, the ball rocketed toward the telephone pole on a straight, unwavering line, took two hops along the same line and bounced up against the pole.

Goose bumps raised along my neck and shoulders. I didn't initially feel a sense of pride; what I had just witnessed seemed merely a statement of fact. I had fully expected to hit my target and, when my goal was accomplished, I wasn't surprised. I decided to repeat the experiment. Again I pictured the ball sailing toward the net, bouncing twice, then hitting off the pole. Again I let the club swing itself, and again my picture was brought to life in my swing. The third time, I pictured the ball bouncing three times before hitting the pole, and I saw the trajectory of my drive being a little higher than before. My shot matched my picture exactly, except, at the last moment, it bounced just to the side of the pole, missing by inches. This felt like a cosmic wink—an assurance that, indeed, I was not in control of this mechanism, *it* was. I became so excited at what had just happened, and at the possibilities that might lie ahead for me in my golf game, that I put down my club and walked over to a pay phone to call my wife to share my excitement with her.

When I told her the story of what I had done, she, too, became excited. She wasn't just happy for me; she could tell that I had come upon something important. She often felt that I didn't believe enough in myself, and she hoped that I had now found a way to be more confident. After listening to me and sharing my excitement, she said to me, "This is wonderful! There are so many things you can do with this. You could even use it in your work."

Her statement jolted me out of my reverie, and annoyed me; she was suggesting that I melt down the key to heaven, and sell it as scrap metal! I wanted to delight in the moment, to share this experience, and look at it as an act of creation; she wanted to know what its use was going to be. "But I'm not talking about my work now," I said, the irritation showing in my voice, "I'm telling you about an experience."

"Yes, but there is so much more you can do with what you've found," she said, almost pleading. "It's not just golf."

I had trouble with those words being put side by side. I became cartoonishly defensive, unreasonable, and arrogant. "Just golf? Just golf? This experience, this moment, *is* golf! When I allow the club to swing itself, golf is everything; there is nothing else."

She realized that she had stepped on my toes, which were often in the way when it came to golf. She knew I was conflicted about playing the game and devoting so much of my attention to it, and she knew that there was no way to get me to see the larger picture of my experience this time. With the deftness of a bullfighter, she stepped gracefully to the side of my oncoming charge. "Well, I didn't mean to rain on your parade." She even resisted her impulse to add, "but there's so much more here," and we hung up.

When I got back to the range, I still was able to hit good shots but, initially, I had the petulant feeling that the wind had been taken out of my sails. I continued to hit balls until again I relaxed into a nice zone. Each shot began to feel crisp again, and I began again to visualize exactly where the ball would go. I started to believe that there was no limitation on how accurate I could be. I could hit any target. Twice, I hit the exact flag I intended to hit. And then something *really* unusual happened: I realized that my wife was right. This wasn't just about golf. If I can visualize what a golf ball will do, then allow that picture to become manifest by swinging a club, what other possibilities are open to me? I fully felt the power of this belief, and again had a strong sense of a presence with me, within me. I wondered what this presence was, and I thought about where I could turn to get answers to the many questions that were coming to me. Had I accessed some kind of natural brain mechanism that allows us to perform our best when we awaken to our potential? The more I thought about these questions, the more I felt I had to follow them wherever they would lead me.

~

MANY GOLFERS HAVE DESCRIBED feeling as if the club is moving on its own. Athletes from other sports have said the same thing. During their epic home run battle in 1998, Sammy Sosa and Mark McGwire independently described a similar experience. McGwire said that, when he was at bat, he sometimes felt as if he had lost control of his body, like he was outside of himself watching in slow motion as the bat connected with the ball perfectly, solidly, creating a force and a power that was generated from outside him.

Years after I first felt that golf club swinging on its own, Dan Brooks, the women's golf coach at Duke, relayed a similar experience when he returned from watching Jenny Chausiriporn play against Se Ri Pak in an eighteen-hole playoff for the 1998 U.S. Women's Open. On the day before the playoff, a group of us who had just played at the Duke University Golf Club watched from the snack bar while Jenny battled to tie Pak. When she made a twisting forty-foot putt to tie for the lead on the 72nd hole—a putt Johnny Miller later described as "the most dramatic putt in the history of the USGA"—the snack bar, filled with middle-aged men and the pro-shop staff, erupted. Several of us were so excited for her (and perhaps wanted so much to latch onto her success) that we looked into hiring a private plane to fly from Durham to Wisconsin to watch the playoff. The Jennymania was eventually nixed since the Duke pro-shop guys would need financial support for the endeavor, and Athletic Director Joe Alleva rightfully decided that would probably violate seventeen different NCAA regulations, as well as three tenets of common sense. The end result, however, was that Dan Brooks got on a plane to fly out to Wisconsin to be there with Jenny. He told me what Jenny had described about her forty-footer on the 72nd hole: "She was so far into the zone that the putter seemed to move on its own." The look of complete shock on her face after she made the putt confirmed that she felt somehow removed from her tremendous achievement.

This experience, associated with a performance so extraordinary that it borders on magic, underscored the importance of the phenomenon. The putter didn't move on its own when she was tapping in for par, which would seem more likely, since tapping in for par is so easy and automatic that the brain could be busy doing something else. No, it moved on its own when this twenty-year-old amateur was standing over the ball peering through the threshold of history. How was it that she and I had had such similar experiences while executing shots that wound up being so phenomenally good? Was this just the way that people overinterpret chance events? Or was there some brain mechanism in operation? What would cause the brain to do this? Was there some adaptive value in parts of the brain dissociating themselves from particular intense experiences? Or were there more specific brain processes involved? The idea that we can be taken over by an outside force that moves our bodies seems highly unlikely but, at this point, I was open to any possibility. And, more than anything, *that* made me feel like I had come upon the right track.

CHAPTER TWO

Follow Your Heart
(The Man of Fess Des Tinny)

GOLF IS HARDLY THE ONLY PLACE in which an athlete can enter this zone. The release of a basketball off the fingers of a wrist snapped perfectly at the absolute apex of the jump and ideal extension of the arm toward the basket: Even if the player were blinded, he would know it was going in. A wide receiver dives at the last moment, having covered fifty yards in five seconds with out-stretched arms converging on a football that occupied a tiny bouncing speck in his visual field when he prepared to dive. Tennis can produce moments of play that exceed everyone's expectations: "How did she get to that?" A full sprint across court culminates with a powerful and graceful sweeping explosion of the racquet through the ball, which hurtles down the line and just nicks the tape. The years of footwork development, strength training, conditioning, and mental preparation combine with the fortuitous shuffling of genes at conception, and all are delivered at the same moment.

The writer John Jerome referred to these athletic moments as "sweet spots in time." The physical and mental development of the athlete, and the event that arises to allow full expression of this development, seem to have been perfectly designed for one another. Golf is full of these events. Even beginners have them. After skimming a bucket's worth of shots across a practice range, the beginning golfer finally makes an adjustment in his swing that lifts the ball into the air, and it bounds past the 150-yard sign. He is delighted, and tries to understand what he did that time to produce that ball flight and feeling of contact with the ball.

Was the beginner's airborne shot skill or chance? Is the tennis player's tremendous get and blast down the line due solely to skill, or is good fortune operating as well? Was my perfectly visualized series of drives on the practice range a function of attaining a perfect approach for that minute, or was I just astronomically lucky to hit the telephone pole repeatedly? Or, do these "sweet spots in time" occur from a burgeoning level of skill relative to previous expectation, combined with peaks of good fortune and a large number of attempts? The beginning golfer may be delighted at getting the ball airborne, and may feel like he is in the zone when he hits consecutive shots past the 150-yard sign. The various fulcrums of his swing may have finally operated in unison for him, and he is better than he was the first time he hit golf balls, but chance is also at work. The hands on a watch will eventually all align in perfect unison at the stroke of noon and midnight. Is there something legitimately special about these moments compared to all the others?

In viewing excellent golf performance as somehow coming from a source outside the self, we may be misinterpreting chance events. After all, gamblers in Las Vegas who are having a string of good luck will frequently say they're "feeling it." Is going into the zone the same as believing that some kind of outside force controls the cards and the dice, so certain gamblers win and others lose? Anyone who frequently engages in any activity can expect at least a few strange occurrences. For people who play a lot of golf, unusual events are almost certain to happen.

Scientist Carl Sagan once discussed the statistics of unusual *precognitive* experiences, in which someone predicts an important event. He had had a vivid dream that his uncle died, and he awoke in a cold sweat, startled and frightened. He felt compelled to call his uncle to check on his premonition; his hypothesis was that his uncle had indeed died, and that he had somehow received a message about the death. Most everyone has heard a story of someone who has had such a precognitive experience. When he called his aunt, she answered the phone and assured him that his uncle was fine and watching television right beside her; he did not die the next day, either. Dr. Sagan noted that he was not moved to write an article for *Psychology Today* in which he described the intensity of the precognitive experience, then the fact that it was totally false. Only when the story is indeed predictive are such stories written. He decided to calculate the chances that someone could successfully predict the death of a close relative. Since most people report having some form of precognitive experience during their lifetime, and many report them quite frequently, a conservative estimate is that on average each person has one per lifetime, which adds up to about three hundred million precognitive experiences across the United States alone. If you assume that any precognitive experience within a week of the death is interesting enough to tell others, then the likelihood is that, by chance, the number of people in the United States who have a precognitive dream about a relative who actually dies is 200 per week! And that doesn't include that fact that people may be more likely to have a precognitive experience about the death if they have some warning that the person was going to die through a chronic illness, or a tendency to drink and drive.

If the number of possible event opportunities is large enough, unusual events are almost certain to happen. People often tell stories of times when someone calls "just as I was thinking of her." Given the number of people we think about over the course of our many days, it seems likely that by chance one of them will call every so often. I probably think about a hundred people per day; some of them I see every day, so a phone call from one of them wouldn't gather a lot of attention. I also think of many people that I haven't seen for years. If I calculate how many people I think of over the course of a year, this adds up to at least 30,000 chances for one of them to call me out of the blue. Something that happens once in 30,000 times is considered a very rare and special event, yet, over the course of a whole year, very rare and special events are statistically *guaranteed* to happen. So, perhaps a coincidental phone call or driving a golf ball off a distant telephone pole repeatedly are really just statistical phenomena that, in the grand scheme of time, are not unusual at all.

~

SOME EVENTS appear so extraordinary that it's difficult for even a statistician to maintain that they were due merely to chance. Furthermore, the greater the personal meaning of the events, the more difficult it is to ascribe them to mere randomness. I had the following experience a few years ago that knocked me right off of my statistical high horse. (I don't like this horse metaphor but, as soon as I typed it, I looked up to see that on the airline movie screen there was a picture of someone high on a horse, viewed from low on the ground. I then felt that perhaps the metaphor was meant to be, so I kept it.)

I was trained in sport psychology by Dick Coop, who has worked with dozens of PGA Tour players, including several prominent players who have won multiple majors. The primary reason I dragged my family down to North Carolina from New Jersey was to be mentored by him as to how to help golfers with the mental side of the game. He had never trained anyone before, yet he was a tremendous teacher; he had somehow chosen me to receive the tools of his trade. I would frequently follow him around as he worked with a golfer; this was relatively easy when he had an amateur player visiting him at the Governor's Club in Chapel Hill, where I would stay a comfortable distance behind him and the golfer and try to be as unobtrusive as possible. None of the golfers seemed to mind my presence.

Maintaining a comfortable following distance was more challenging at PGA Tour events. While even Dick wasn't allowed inside the ropes that protected the course from spectators during the actual tournament, there are many other cordoned-off areas that are accessible to teachers whose players had them sanctioned by the PGA Tour. There is a clear division between those who are a part of the show and those who are watching: Dick was a part of the show, albeit the supporting cast, while I could best be described as a hanger-on. At the first Tour event I attended with Dick, we arrived on the Wednesday before the tournament started. One of his players was the defending champion, and was the center of attention during the pro-am. The player was very friendly to me, referring to me as Dick's "prodigy," and he encouraged me to join the group walking with him as he played. Later, Dick brought me with him onto the putting green while he worked with the current National Champion on his putting. I felt clumsy, like a voyeur or a groupie, yet it was fun to pretend that I belonged, and I appreciated Dick including me fully in his world. The warmth that the Tour players felt toward Dick was clear, and they readily accepted me, even if I was having trouble feeling like I fit in.

Thursday of the tournament was different. When the first round started, the great increase in the number of spectators brought an increase in security, and the informal, all-access pass I'd had yesterday was suddenly severely limited. Although I had felt awkward being inside the ropes, suddenly being shut out of the practice areas and clubhouse was far worse. While Dick went in to eat with his players and talk to them about their rounds, I had to wait outside like everyone else, no longer special. That first year, I made the most of it: I sat and talked with caddies a bit, studied some of the players' practice routines, or walked the course watching the *action*, a term whose usage is fully stretched when applied to tournament golf. I also stood behind the fence at the practice range watching Dick work with his players. I felt that I learned a lot from the experience, and I enjoyed having been included for a while, if only to be eventually pushed back into my usual spot.

A year later, after having worked with Dick for almost two full years, I began to have a different attitude about going to a tournament. Dick had taught me extensively how to work with golfers in general, and we had focused a lot on the special circumstances of working with players on the PGA Tour. This second year of being prohibited from going certain places at a Tour event became wearing. As much as I appreciated Dick's efforts to include me, my attendance at the tournament felt too much like a fan rubbing elbows with Tour players. I was training to work with golfers as part of my profession, and I had a growing sense that I could offer something even to those at the top levels of their profession. I guess I wanted to be involved in the show.

One Monday, after having gone to three days of a PGA Tour event with Dick, I picked up a goal-setting workbook that a friend had designed. While looking it over, I realized that, while I'd been spending a lot of time helping others to set and reach their goals, I hadn't really set any goals for myself. I had felt that I wasn't ready yet, and I hadn't considered what I wanted to be headed toward. As I thought this over that morning, I went about my usual business of preparing to go to my office. While in the shower, I very distinctly set a course: I felt that working with a PGA Tour player would perhaps be a little overwhelming at this stage, but that working with a player at golf's version of the triple-A minor leagues, at the time called the Nike Tour, would be perfect. That would be my goal. I saw it happening. By the time my shower was over, I felt a certainty about my next step on this journey. I had no idea at this point of how

I'd achieve this goal; I felt that the details would somehow work themselves out. It was a strange, blind faith, but I believed in my vision with absolutely no reason to do so. I headed off for work happy and inspired.

When I got to my office, some thirty minutes later, my secretary handed me a message that my wife, Caren, had called, and that I should call home immediately. Caren told me that, a few minutes after I'd left the house, a player from the Nike Tour had called me. He had gone to his college coach to talk about some of the difficulties he'd been having with his confidence and concentration, and his coach told him that he should start working with me.

How did this process work? How was I transformed sequentially from being rudderless in my beginning career in sport psychology to seeing a clear vision snap into focus to having that goal achieved almost instantaneously? Was this just an unbelievable and fortunate coincidence? Did the image of what I wanted, ignored for months, if not years, then brought into light, have an actual impact on the outside world? I had not prayed for this outcome, but was this the same cosmic mechanism at work—ask and you shall receive? Or were there signs all around that I was about to have this opportunity, but I didn't see them until the very last moment before the goal was achieved? The sequence of events floored me. Better still, the opportunity bore fruit: The player and I really connected, and the relationship enhanced both our careers. While he had had only one top ten finish in the first half of the season before we began working together, by the time the season was over he had won twice, barely missing qualifying for the PGA Tour.

This series of events could be considered a precognitive success story: I had a vision, and it was almost immediately realized. However, only the match between the outcome and the prediction makes the story worth telling. How many stories of mismatches between prediction and outcome are told? Very few: "I had a strong premonition that I would meet my future wife that day. But, as usual, I went home alone." This sequence of events is so typical that it's not worth relaying to anybody. The vast majority of our predictions never come true, and we quickly forget them; we remember the ones that came true because they grab our attention. Research shows that we remember events better if our emotions are increased in relation to them, and we are far more likely to generate emotion about an unusual successful prediction than we are about the banal premonition that misses the target.

Post hoc explanations are particularly suspect. If an unusual event occurs, then, after struggling to understand it, we ascribe its occurrence to some sort of universal consciousness or cosmic force, the explanatory power of this conclusion is fairly weak. Humans have a remarkable tendency to make sense out of nonsense. Studies of research professors in the behavioral sciences have demonstrated this in an exaggerated form: When asked to interpret data that were actually a series of random numbers, the professors derived all kinds of complex and clever explanations for what was essentially meaningless information. The facility of some neuroscientists to develop *post hoc* explanations of their data is impressive. Since some neural systems inhibit certain brain functions, and other neural systems *disinhibit* these functions, it is always possible to interpret data as suggesting inhibition or disinhibition of function. When told that he had not noticed the minus sign in front of the correlations he was discussing, the neuroscience professor did not skip a beat: "Oh, very interesting, these neurons must be having a *disinhibitory* effect, not an inhibitory one." Many of us act and think in our daily lives much like the professor backed into a corner by an incisive question during his scientific presentation: There is a complete inability to place in sequence the words *I, don't,* and *know.*

I quite literally saw a chicken cross a road the other day, right in front of my oncoming car. It had wandered away from its home toward a swamp on the other side of the road. I don't think that the chicken was interested in the other side. I don't really know why it crossed the road. I suspect that chickens, like humans, have a basic tendency to keep moving. Movement keeps the biological systems healthy and functioning well. Sometimes the movement *is* the purpose, whether it's the legs of a chicken away from the coop, or the meandering calculations of our desire to explain the world around us. The place at which our journey ends, however, may be no more meaningful than the place at which it began.

By now, you may be thinking that I'm completely devoid of romance and adventure, wanting only to see cold facts, even in an instance when the outside world has been so warm to me. However, I greatly value intuition, and believe there are some mechanisms in the brain and, perhaps, in the universe, that increase the chances that our intuitions will be expressed in the external world. But, I want to see this mechanism for what it really is, not what I sometimes want it to be.

The development of real intuition is complex and circuitous. My attempts to understand it have often been fruitless: I am certain that I will hole a 120-foot chip, and I do. How did this certainty come to be? Am I really able to know the future based upon some kind of semiconscious, in-depth analysis? I've sometimes focused on this question throughout an entire round of golf, determining my degree of certainty that I would make a putt, then observing the percentage of the time that I was correct. I've also noticed that, when I approach the putt as an objective experiment in this way—"let's see if the intuition works this time"—it almost always fails. I first thought that this justified my skepticism, since my failure to hole the putt would come at a time when I was doubting the certainty I'd felt. Then, I realized that my objectivity was not neutral; it was skeptical and, as such, it confounded my little experiment. My state of mind was the independent measure, the experimental manipulation, so it was an experiment that I could not actually conduct. I was either fully in the moment of my shot, allowing my certainty to rise and following the image that it had created, or I was outside myself, observing scientifically; only in retrospect could I determine whether I was fully in the present or whether I was objective and skeptical. This retrospective view of my action is dramatically colored by the result: I'm more likely to amplify my perception of how certain I was prior to the putt if I actually hole it (the putt goes in: "I knew it was going in!") and minimize it if it misses (the putt misses: "I was skeptical on that one.") It is impossible to get an objective view of this subjective process; we either trust the shot or we don't and, the more we trust, the better we seem to do.

Archie Miller, a North Carolina State point guard who led the NCAA in three-point percentage before suffering an injury in 2000, said that he could feel the difference between being in a zone and not. "Sometimes I'll make three in a row, and don't feel like I'm in the zone at all; other times, I'll hit a couple and then it's like, 'oh, here it comes.' " Perhaps one of the attributes of the most successful athletes is being able to recognize when to just sit back and let the effortless excellence emanate from the center of their being.

It may also be that our beliefs in what is true and our use of beliefs for getting the results we want are different. I had had a vision of working with a Nike Tour player; one called out of the blue, within an hour. It makes me feel good to believe that there is a mechanism in the universe that supports my wants and guides me toward greater things. Not knowing what this mechanism is, or not understanding how it works, shouldn't stop me from letting it enrich my life.

~

I RAISED THE SUBJECT of these types of coincidence with a close friend of mine, Jeff Kennedy. Jeff is a levelheaded dentist whom I've known since we were ten years old. He went to Duke, met his future wife there, and the two of them stayed in the area; when my family and I moved to North Carolina, one of the things I looked forward to was being able to share our experiences of being fathers and husbands. He is very bright, yet practical and skeptical. When I began discussing the ideas I'd been having about coincidences and premonition, Jeff was very interested, and had a number of theories on the phenomena. After we talked about that subject for a while, we somehow wound up discussing the Just Say No substance abuse prevention program. I had heard that the whole effort had been very successful, and we were both surprised that it had, yet we were happy that fewer kids were using drugs than in the past. "It's nice that it's working; I hope it keeps helping through our kids' time," he said. As soon as he finished his sentence, the phone rang. Jeff politely declined to donate money to the organization that was calling. *More polite than I usually am,* I thought.

"Who was it?" I asked.

"Just Say No," he answered with no hint of irony on his face.

"You're kidding, right?" I asked.

"No, why?" he answered.

He hadn't made the connection between our discussion of the Just Say No organization and their simultaneous call, even though we'd been discussing our mutual interest in these types of coincidences just a few minutes before! At that point, it occurred to me that there is also a powerful tendency among some of us not to highlight these types of experiences. I don't know why. Do we deny the experiences, or does this ascribe too much will to our limitations? Perhaps we are just not trained to see them and to utilize our abilities.

~

A COLLEAGUE ONCE SAID TO ME, "There are two kinds of people: those who dichotomize, and those who don't." This pressure to create a world of this *versus* that affects the way we see chance and intuition. "Is it one . . . or the other?" It is probably not this simple.

Humans have the capacity to interpret even the faintest signal in the noisiest background. We are constantly flooded with stimuli from at least three of our five senses, and we're usually very good at picking out what's relevant to us. Right now, you are not only reading these words, but hearing some kind of background noise (if not, your startled brain has created for you a faint ringing in your ears) and, if you attend to your body, you will feel the book in your hand and the pull of gravity in the contact of your skin to your chosen resting place. You may even be struggling with odors and tastes, foul or sweet. We take these abilities for granted, yet they are almost unfathomably complex. Living things have the ability to interpret some of the electromagnetic frequencies that are present on this planet, such as audible sound and visible light, but these form a very narrow window of the broad range of available frequencies. Just think how difficult life would be if we were able to perceive radio frequencies or microwaves.

In the same way in which we select what is important to us from a chaotic rapture of sound waves and electromagnetic noise, we often find a pattern of logical relationships in a haystack of chance events. Like our ability to perceive, our logical understanding of the world around us helps us to survive. Our five senses are very impressive indeed, but what about this *sixth* one? Some people are highly attuned to such possibilities; they look at you with raised and knowing eyebrows at every little chance coincidence. My gregarious mother-in-law is the poster child for this segment of the population; after having survived a lifetime with my father-in-law's lack of interest in other people, every moment for her may seem miraculous. Others turn their sensitivity down very low or off altogether; even the greatest coincidences are shrugged off with an "interesting," that serves only to end the discussion. In the middle of this spectrum, however, lies the possibility of a more complex and intriguing relationship between intuition and chance.

An elevated certainty about future events, such as a prescient image of making a putt, may come from an increase in information, suddenly available to us, that we did not know we possessed. We see the line perfectly, and develop a certainty that we know exactly what the roll will be like, what stroke and speed are required. We have accessed more information than usual, and a part of our brain knows that.

Suppose that I see something in the newspaper that reminds me of a friend. The friend also sees the same thing in his newspaper across the country and is reminded of me. Later that day, when I am still thinking of him from time to time, he calls; I don't connect his calling with the newspaper story and he doesn't either, so the event seems like a magical coincidence. However, it was an event that was predetermined by both of us having more information than we realized that we had. My friend Jeff and I may have been talking about the Just Say No group because one of us had read a newspaper article discussing their new phone soliciting campaign, though we had forgotten about that trigger. The connection seemed magical because we had lost awareness of the connection between the events. Regarding the high-horse metaphor that seemed to have been supported by universal destiny in the form of an airline movie screen, maybe I had previously seen another horse on the screen without being aware of it, which led to the metaphor in the first place. The negative side of this discussion is that we often overinterpret the presence of a guiding universal force in our lives; that's not to say that there isn't one, just that we see it in places where it is not. The positive side is that we seem to underestimate our highly developed evolutionary ability to guide ourselves where we really want to go.

If there is a greater intuition or a higher awareness available to us, how can we gain more frequent access to it? That day at the driving range, I may have somehow become aware that I was about to reach the peak of my skill and accuracy with my driver. I thus set out to sit back and experience this heightened level of skill, which let it spring out of me. My true premonition may have been that I had accessed a trust in myself. I had realized that I would be able to do something extraordinary, and I found the mechanism to reduce my real-world doubt. I allowed the club to swing itself. My realism did not inhibit the leap toward a new level of ability that I'd sensed I had attained.

~

DRIVING HOME FROM Jeff's house, after having been struck by this very attentive man's lack of attention to the coincidence of the Just Say No phone call, I wondered whether there is a way to aid the development of this type of intuition. I recalled a game my father played with me, called *follow your heart*. Most Saturday mornings, when I was about five or six, he would take me out for a drive or, more accurately, I would take him out for a drive. There were only two rules: I told him where to drive, but I wasn't allowed to choose a direction if I knew why I chose it as in, "Turn here, Dad, down this road is Playtown Park!" The other rule was that we weren't allowed to disobey traffic signs so, sometimes, I'd tell him to go down a one-way street, and he would tell me I had to try again. It seemed we always wound up someplace that was fun in a way that was unique. We often found parks and jungle gyms I never knew existed. I assumed that my father didn't know where we were headed either, since he seemed surprised by some of the places at which we arrived. He always spoke about our destination as though it were fulfilling a want or a need of mine. Sometimes he referred to our final destination grandly as our "Manifest Destiny," which I pronounced "Man of Fess Des Tinny," and thought it was the name of a mysterious man who lived long ago in a foreign-sounding land. Although my father emphasized that we were fulfilling *my* vision, I remember feeling that this man from Fess Des Tinny was helping guide me to a special place. I didn't realize it at the time, and I don't think my father was considering it this way, but he was training me to cultivate a sort of higher awareness. These drives were really lessons about the potential of the brain to lead itself unconsciously through a complex world. I was learning to trust my heart, my intuition, even before my logic had developed.

I have recently begun playing this game again. My children enjoy it as I did, and I love passing on to them this trust in themselves. I have also noticed that the process still leads me to things that I could never have expected, yet am delighted to find. I even take walks like this on my own when I'm traveling on business; each turn is guided not by logic, but by a feeling that allowing this higher consciousness to guide me will benefit me somehow. Sometimes, I wind up helping someone I've come across; other times, I meet and interact with a native of the area. It seems to be an especially effective way to select a restaurant in a city where I've never been. Perhaps this is why men refuse to stop the car to ask for directions: We prefer to follow our hearts.

It was no coincidence that I thought of my father in the context of developing intuition. Trust is not easy to come by in a world rich with threats to our survival. If we're taught in our childhood to fear the chance occurrences life brings us, we'll carry that fear through to our grave. If we're taught to have faith that these events will provide for us, our steps past the graveyard will be light.

Early relationships are important in building trust in one's golf game. How an adult–child relationship progresses on the golf course is especially important, as it will certainly affect how the child learns to trust her golf, and how she grows to believe in herself in general. If we're criticized for poor shots while we're learning the game, we'll later approach each shot with an image of that potential criticism.

Since the social pressures of golf are high, criticism regarding the outcome of a shot runs parallel with many other objects of our self-consciousness, such as our pace of play or how we look. For a child learning golf, these issues may all fuse together in a vague mass of nervousness and, as any golfer knows, this type of anxiety makes us play worse. It also makes us live worse. Constant attention to an external view of oneself is the core of human angst. If we could think of disastrous shots as one unfortunate possibility in a pleasant pastime, we would be better able to enjoy the challenge of the moment. Further, feeling trust in a golf shot opens up the door for learning how to trust ourselves in other aspects of life. So, each round with a child is literally a growth opportunity: Will we fill it with bitter lessons in how he or she fails to measure up to our adult expectations? Or will it be filled with lessons of faith in himself or herself, and a connection to the adult who was trusting and patient in the face of adversity? As with an ally in a war, a buddy in a bunker, that kind of bond can last through the decades.

An amateur golfer who came to me to for a consultation told me that, when he began to trust his intuition and fall into the zone on the golf course, he had frequent vivid memories of his father, and began thinking of him often, even off the golf course. His father had died about twenty years earlier and, although the golfer had some vague memories of having grieved when he died, he did not remember giving his father a tremendous amount of thought. He had learned from his mother recently, however, that, when he was nine years old, he was so crushed and distraught at his father's funeral, that he tried to climb into the coffin to be with him. In retrospect, he realized that he had become increasingly serious and pragmatic after his father died. He found himself unable to trust people, and even small slights were devastating. His relationships with women were punctuated by his intense criticism of their most minor faults, as though each blemish revealed the hidden truth about their inadequacy. At the core of his problems with other people was his complete inability to trust his own judgment. It was as though the little boy who had developed intuition in the presence of his father died with his father and only when he started to trust himself on the golf course did that part of him come to life again. He described to me an image he had of a bright, alert, and irritated young boy emerging from his father's coffin, pushing aside his father's corpse and saying to him, "Finally! Can I come back out again?"

~

Is THERE A DELIBERATE WAY to become sensitive to this greater awareness in golf and other sports? How do we turn up the gain on our intuition receiver, without adding noise? I will discuss this issue in later chapters from several perspectives. When people come to me for advice regarding a difficult decision, after weighing all the options they usually have a gut feeling that they really want to follow. It seems like a simple exercise, and it's strange to them that they weren't aware of the strength of this gut feeling before I've asked them to access it. Talking to someone else who is really listening seems to give us the courage to move toward our intuition. So does remembering someone who believed in us, or believes in us, or a time when we fully trusted ourselves. In the presence of someone who appears to be on our side, our self-doubt is weakened and our trust in ourselves can emerge. A good caddie helps a player develop confidence in the club choice the player wanted to make all along.

Talking helps us trace our opinions; by hearing ourselves think and feel, we can burrow through complex, conflicting emotions to reach a clearer understanding of the deeper recesses of our hearts. By being encouraged, we lose our fear. And, when we lose our fear, we gravitate toward our true being without restraint. We follow our hearts to our manifest destiny.

CHAPTER THREE

Neurons Reaching
Toward Faith

S O FAR, WE'VE CONSIDERED the possibilities that chance and intuition explain my experience of the club swinging itself and the resulting exceptional performance. I now want to look at what neurobiology can teach us about how the brain allows such an experience, and why this type of brain function may be important in our everyday lives.

At the time I had that experience, I knew very little about the brain; although I've now studied it intensively for several years, the amount that I do not know far outweighs the amount I have learned, and this ratio only worsens with time. New data emerge almost every week, and our findings suggest that the brain is more complex, more flexible, and more adaptive than anyone had ever considered.

When I arrived at Duke in 1995, I had just received a research grant to study how the brain is impaired in people with schizophrenia, so I had a good excuse to learn how the brain is activated by basic mental operations. Some of these lessons allowed me to study the initiation of motor activity, which I felt would shed light on the brain mechanisms behind my experiences.

One of the first conversations I had on this topic was with Dr. Roland Perlmutter, a neuroradiologist at Duke University Medical Center. Roland was a short and somewhat handsome man. His head was larger than most, and he was so bright that, upon meeting him, I had the impression that his brain was just different from the rest of ours. I had initially contacted Roland to discuss a potential collaboration on a schizophrenia brain-imaging project. However, I also wanted to find out from him what was going on in *my* brain—what were the neurological implications of the experiences I was having? The most striking aspect of meeting Roland was the certainty he seemed to feel about everything he told me. At first, I found this arrogance boorish. However, since I was feeling a great deal of uncertainty about what had been happening to me at the time, his certainty about his opinions became somehow reassuring.

After discussing our potential schizophrenia research together, our conversation moved to the topic of my experiences. After listening intently to my story about my frequent feeling that the golf club was swinging on its own, he got very excited and exclaimed, "Fabulous! The effortless present!" He walked over to a computer with a liquid crystal monitor that was extra tall and wide, but only one inch thick. At the time, I had never before seen a monitor like this. He clicked on a small icon of a brain, and it exploded into a life-size picture of an axial slice of a human brain, cut back to front as though the top half of the person's head had been removed. "This is your brain," he said, pointing to the vivid black-and-white picture that looked like a high-resolution x ray, except this one also had red and blue splotches on it. "Well, obviously it's not *your* brain, but it could be— it's the brain of one of our volunteers who has nothing wrong. Now, here's one from someone with damage to a particular part of their frontal lobes."

He clicked on the icon of a different brain. The red splotches, which indicated that the brain was very active, were almost nonexistent in the top part of the image, where the frontal lobes are located.

"Do you see how the normal brain has so much activity in the frontal lobes, while the one with brain damage has almost nothing going on there?"

I had seen imaging data numerous times before, but I was proud that I was able to follow along so far. This Perlmutter wasn't going to try to just overwhelm me with how much he knew; rather, he was going to teach me. I began to feel a sense of relief and anticipation that some of my questions had answers, and Perlmutter was about to give them to me.

"That's pretty consistent with what we know about this type of brain damage," he said. "We asked people to observe themselves moving their fingers and, even though all the patients with frontal lobe damage could do what we asked with no problem, the parts of the normal brain that are monitoring the movement, right here, were completely silent in the patients. We expected this, because we chose patients who have experiences that are a part of something called *wayward hand syndrome*. They occasionally have these weird experiences that an external force is moving their limbs or their bodies. So, it makes sense that they would not activate the parts of their brain that normally monitor the initiation of their movements. But here is where it gets exciting, especially for you: Some professional piano players have the same pattern of activation as the patients with frontal lobe damage—they don't appear to be monitoring the initiation of their movements. Their frontal cortex doesn't activate at all when they move their fingers. The movement is regulated by other, more basic, parts of the brain, like their motor cortex or even their cerebellum."

His connection to musicians was interesting, but I was afraid he was going to move away from the topic, as some academicians are wont to do. I had once attended a conference on brain imaging in which some of the speakers discussed the brain activation associated with mastery. One of them discussed her data suggesting that piano players had brain structure and function that were different from those who had never played. The topic had intrigued me at the time, but its relevance to sport wasn't immediately obvious to me. "What do piano player studies have to do with my experiences?" I asked.

"Well, you have to keep your head perfectly still in the scanner, otherwise the brain images won't register properly. And since you have to be lying down, making a golf swing is impossible, so we can't really study golfers swinging a golf club, but we can understand them and other athletes by analogy. The largest amount of movement we can allow without disrupting the data collection is tapping your fingers. And who are expert finger tappers? Piano players and typists. It turns out that piano players are better to study since they have usually been doing it since they were little children, which actually changes the way the brain is formed. Besides, with piano players, the best ones are easy to find. We image the piano players just as they are about to initiate action. For you, this would be when you are over the ball and are just about to bring the club back. Have you ever noticed that most Tour players spend very little time at this stage? Once they're over the ball, they go ahead and initiate the swing. The beginning player takes forever over the ball because he's still trying to figure out what to do. The beginner's mind is a jumble of conflicting motor programs. The Tour player just sits back and lets it go."

I was stunned that Perlmutter also knew about golf. I found myself becoming passive and attentive, almost like I was in the audience of a tremendously absorbing film.

"This brief period of time is the most important part of any deliberate action: just prior to its initiation," he went on. "It's crucial in many sports: sprinters awaiting the starting gun, basketball players about to shoot foul shots, tennis players preparing to serve or return a serve. The piano players are able to perform their expert function without attention to the initiation of the movement. When they play the piano, their experience is that the music just flows out of them. They are thinking about the sounds they want to produce, and their hands just move as if on their own; they give no thought at all to how their fingers should move or how to form a particular chord—it feels to them as though the movement is just unfolding in front of them. I call it 'the effortless present.' They describe it as very pleasant, even ecstatic, sometimes."

I waited for Perlmutter to continue, even though he had clearly completed his side of what had once been a conversation. Perlmutter seemed not to be affected by the long pause in our conversation resulting from my withdrawal; I surmised that he was used to saying things that left people speechless and pondering. He had moved on to other things, however, and pulled out a form for me to complete and sign if I wanted to volunteer for his research study. He raised his eyebrows in a flirtatious way. "Do you want to be a subject in our latest experiment?" he asked. "I think you'll find it interesting."

"Sure," I said, as Perlmutter led me toward the scanner, which looked like a nine-foot-high donut with a table coming out of the hole. I lay down on the table, and it began sliding me into the center of the scanner. Once I was situated, the whole process took about an hour. First, my brain structure was recorded, then I completed Dr. Perlmutter's finger-movement task, which was very simple. The sounds that the machine made during the experiment were bizarre, from loud clanging and pounding to a strange whooping sound. I had to wear earplugs to minimize the noise. I tried to ignore the sounds and just lie back and respond to the pictures of hands that were appearing on the screen, directing me which fingers to move. Some of the more complex finger movements required more attention and effort, while others were very simple and effortless. The simpler movements seemed to flow out of me like a smooth nine-iron or a perfectly struck downhill putt. When I was finished with the experiment in the scanner, Perlmutter analyzed the data that had been collected from my brain, revealing colored splotches where my brain had been particularly active. He seemed impressed with my brain.

"I have a hypothesis that some of the reduced frontal activation we see in the piano players is not specific to playing piano—that people who are able to experience the zone in their athletic activity can reduce their frontal activation at will. This may be the mechanism that separates great players from the rest in any sport; they can stop monitoring their movements and just let them happen on their own regardless of what the movements are, as long as they are relatively simple or practiced. You seem to fit this pattern."

I was flattered and excited, and leaned over to get a better view of my brain activation. I could see some brightly lit areas in the middle of the brain, and some unlit areas in the frontal part. I felt strangely proud of my brain, and had a brief idea that I was special in some way, which immediately made me anxious. As I often did, I interrupted my feelings of being impressed with myself by saying something stupid: I pointed to one of the brightly lit sections of my brain and said, "I think, therefore I am."

Perlmutter laughed politely, then shook his head bemusedly. "Those old coots like Descartes, saying stuff like 'I think, therefore I am,' they didn't know anything about the brain. When Descartes referred to *thinking* he was only referring to the tip of the iceberg in terms of brain function. We are performing a hundred mental operations without being aware, or without thinking of what we are doing. You know, like the *cocktail-party phenomenon.*"

(The *cocktail-party phenomenon* is an everyday demonstration of our ability to attend to several things at once, even though we are not aware of all of them. Imagine you are at a party, and you are listening attentively to the person with whom you're conversing; if someone were to ask you about any of the other conversations in the room, you'd probably have no idea what they were about. However, if someone across the room said something that you were particularly interested in, like your name, you'd hear it and shift your attention that way. Essentially, your brain is staying open to all of the other conversations at the same time, searching for anything that might be relevant or interesting to you, but you are pretty much unaware of it; only when the search mechanism finds something important is your attention shifted toward it. There are many aspects of your internal and external world that are processed continuously, yet don't enter your awareness until you need them.

A crude way to relate the cocktail-party phenomenon to the functional division in the brain is that the cortex, which means *bark*, like the bark of a tree, because it's the outermost layer of the brain, is the part of the brain involved in a lot of the things we are aware of, while the *subcortex*, that is, the inner parts of the brain beneath the bark, are involved in a lot of the basic activities that only get our attention when something basic is wrong, like breathing, hunger, staying balanced, and so on.)

Perlmutter continued, "Unless you meditate, you probably only pay attention to your breath when it becomes labored due to something like physical exertion, being underwater, or standing behind an idling bus. Yet the subcortical regions of your brain are constantly attending to your breath—keeping it going, adjusting when necessary, making sure that everything is okay. Of course, the cortical regions can also do a lot of things that we are unaware of, but it's a little more complicated. If I'm a pacifist and you make me so angry that I want to kill you, that intention may be unacceptable to me. So, I can stay unaware of it forever, unless I find myself stalking you with a loaded weapon in my hand. There are also a lot of things we're unaware of that are not just deep forbidden impulses, but truths."

I felt a slight nervousness when he said this, a vague uneasiness somewhere between my chest and belly. I knew he was about to say something important, and I was afraid that I wouldn't be able to understand it. I gave a face of listening very intently and tried to concentrate, but now I was engaged in a three-part task of attention: minding his words and meaning, attempting to look attentive and involved, and also focusing on my worries about whether I would understand him. The difference between listening and being worried that I would not understand was perceptible and annoying. It occurred to me that listening to Perlmutter should come with an FDA warning: talking with this man may produce intestinal cramping; wait thirty minutes after eating before initiating conversation.

"Truths?" I asked, playing for time so that I could batten down the hatches to await the storm of information that was sure to wash over me.

"Yes. Truths! I saw a presentation of a study from the Damasio group in Iowa. I think the paper is being reviewed in *Science.*" (The paper was published in the journal *Science* in 1997.)

I had not heard of the study, but thought that I should have, since *Science* is probably the most respected scientific journal in the world, and I was being paid to do this kind of research.

"Well," he said, "they developed this gambling task and gave it to healthy people and to people who had had damage to the ventromedial aspect of their frontal cortex. That part of the brain is about an inch or so deep right in there," and he pointed directly to the middle lower part of my forehead, about where some people talk about feeling their *third eye.*

"The task was like this: The subjects were given a pile of two thousand dollars in play money and told they should try to make as much money as they could during the experiment. They were to choose cards from four different decks. The cards told them whether they lost money or made money. If the card said something like –*$50*, then fifty dollars was taken from their pile; if it said +*$50*, then fifty dollars was added to their pile. Their level of anxiety was measured by something called *skin-response conductance*, which was simply an electrode attached to their arm. It gave the experimenters an idea of when the subjects were nervous during the test. What the subjects did not know was that two of the decks were *good* decks and two of them were *bad* decks. The good cards offered small winnings and small losses, but overall would result in more money in their pile. The bad cards offered large winnings and large losses, and overall would result in money being taken from their pile. The point of the experiment was to see when the subjects became aware that the good decks earned them money and the bad decks lost them money, and whether their skin response suggested that they knew which decks were good and bad before they were *aware* that they knew. The experimenters asked them every ten cards whether they had developed a strategy for choosing the cards, and related their answers to their deck choices and their anxiety as measured by their skin response."

"So, the researchers were trying to find out if people knew before they knew they knew?" I asked, awkwardly.

"Exactly!" he exclaimed. "And that is precisely what happened. In fact, I think the title of the article is 'Deciding Advantageously Before Knowing the Advantageous Strategy.' Most of the healthy subjects didn't realize until card eighty that there were financially advantageous and disadvantageous decks of cards, yet by card fifty, they started to avoid the decks that lost them money. The most interesting part of the study to me, though, was that the skin response index of anxiety started lighting up when they pulled a card from the bad decks—by card 10! Even though they were initially more likely to sort to the bad decks because they were impressed by the large occasional winnings, they got anxious doing it. Then, later, they began avoiding the bad decks even though when they were asked if there was a pattern, they had no idea! So, as you said before, they knew before they knew they knew.

"The patients with damage to their frontal cortex were much different from the other, healthy subjects. Half of them never were able to figure out that the bad decks would lose them money. The other half figured it out, and were able to describe it to the experimenters, yet they never stopped sorting to the bad decks, and the bad decks didn't make them anxious! So, this part of the frontal cortex, the ventromedial part, seems to be involved not only in helping us figure out what's dangerous and what's safe and advantageous, but it also helps us act on what we unconsciously know to be true, even if we are not aware that it is right. We probably use this part of our brain all the time without really being aware of it. You know the feeling of having a hunch, right? You know in your heart that something is true, even though all the logical evidence is to the contrary. And the stronger you feel that thing to be true, no matter how outlandish, the more likely it is to actually be true, right? Well, that's your ventromedial frontal cortex! It's not your heart, it's your ventromedial frontal cortex!" he exclaimed with a chuckle, his eyes looking at me intensely and his head tilted to one side as if to invite a brilliant response from me, which was not forthcoming.

I thought of all the poems that would have to be revised due to this research. I envisioned my future grandson proposing marriage to a young woman, down on one knee, "Darling, I love you completely and I know we are meant to be together. I feel it deep within my ventromedial cortex." How romantic.

I was suddenly hit by the memory of my father's Saturday game, *follow your heart.* Perlmutter was doing research on what my father had believed in years ago. What had happened to all the training in trusting myself that my father had given me? I often had hunches, often felt that I knew something to be true, yet I hesitated to act because I was afraid of being wrong, of being foolish, maybe of being who I really am. Usually I would postpone doing something long enough to figure out why my hunch was wrong. I had always thought this was my healthy skepticism, but Perlmutter was suggesting that I had learned to ignore an important part of my brain, perhaps even deactivated it. I had a memory of my leg coming out of a cast when I was younger: It was tiny and flabby, and compared to my other leg, looked more like an old woman's arm. Could my ventromedial frontal cortex have atrophied similarly?

Almost on cue, Perlmutter addressed my question before I had asked it. This time, though, he was not reassuring. "I've heard some scientific gossip that Elizabeth Gould from Princeton may have found evidence that the primate brain can generate new neurons. If this is true, it may be that when people begin to use a part of their brain a lot, brain cells may be generated selectively in that area. If they don't use that area much, it actually may get smaller. Most brain functions are mediated by a vast array of neuronal connections, called a *network*; the more a particular network is activated, the faster and stronger the electrochemical messages pass through it. We're still not sure how it works, but there may be a substance, or a bunch of substances, that are released when the network is active, and these substances generate growth of the neurons or, at least, growth in the connections between neurons of certain networks. If you look at this system at the level of two connected brain cells, an increase in the frequency with which they communicate leads to an increase in the substance that gets each of them to grow and develop new connections in the same area. At the level of the whole brain, this growth process results in the brain being able to recognize that a particular activity is important, and then to direct its growth toward the networks and brain areas that are the most active. This is how the adage 'practice makes perfect' really works: The more you do something, the more the brain changes to devote its energy to that function.

"The latest research suggests something that we never suspected: If you practice a particular movement a lot, like the same finger-tapping sequence every day for twenty minutes, the network of neurons that regulates that movement will change dramatically. The areas most associated with thinking about the movement, such as the frontal cortex, will become more active at first, as though increased energy is required to perfect the movement. Then these areas become less active—as if they're no longer necessary. The areas that are responsible for the movement, such as the motor cortex or even the cerebellum, become more active over time—they seem to develop the capacity to regulate the movement all by themselves. It's an unbelievably efficient little system. The brain seems to be wired to understand that if some kind of movement is important and needs attention, the brain areas that monitor that movement will increase their activation, as if the brain is saying 'Uh-oh, we're doing this activity a lot; it must be important. We'd better move in some reinforcements.' Then, when the activity is practiced repeatedly, the network of neurons becomes very efficient at performing the action, and the additional brain activation is no longer needed. Like in a war, when a region is involved in a constant battle, there are frequent lines of communication with the officers and generals; when the region has been conquered and the area is stable, the commanding officers turn their attention somewhere else. So, the area that monitors the initiation of the movement activates fewer neurons, and the person who's doing the moving begins to experience the movement as automatic. The movement actually isn't automatic, it's just that the parts of the brain that need to pay attention to the initiation of action become so deactivated that the rest of the brain—what we call our *self*—doesn't perceive any activity at all."

At the time, much of this research was new to me, and I was a bit confused. Perlmutter's casual mention of the *self* made me think that he was going to enter a whole new discussion that was going to make my head hurt. I decided to try to postpone that conversation for another time. "I think I understand," I said, "but I thought that more is better in the brain—the more activity in an area, the better it performs the movement associated with that region."

"Well, it's complicated, and I don't want to tell you that we know things that haven't been worked out yet. Bigger is certainly better for some functions. For instance, the size of people's hippocampi is strongly correlated with how good their memory is. Yet, for other functions, particularly those that have several components—like a golf swing—the network that mediates them will become more active in some areas and less active in others as performance improves. It's really the network that's key; if you can understand how brain functions are mediated by networks, then you can understand how repeated practice can actually reduce the activation of part of the network: the function is embedded in each aspect of the network. If you want to move your finger, this movement is mediated by a network that includes a series of incredibly strong connections between the cerebellum . . ." (he cupped his hand against the back of his head indicating the location of this brain area as a basketball referee would make a charging call) ". . . which is connected to the finger movement area in the motor cortex . . ." (he indicated this area by pointing halfway between the front and back of his head and about two-thirds of the way down from the top of his head to his ear) ". . . which is connected to the supplementary motor area, in the middle of your brain about an inch forward of that" (he then moved his finger over to the middle of his head and an inch forward) ". . . this area initiates the movement; and the frontal cortex that monitors the initiation of the movement is here" (he moved his finger to the third-eye spot in the middle of his forehead). "As this network is grown and fortified, the initiation of the movement will be so strongly connected to the movement itself that the cells responsible for initiation will hardly need to be activated. The movement will be experienced as occurring on its own because the monitoring system received no signal from the movement-initiation neurons. Look at our muscles as an analogy: Who devotes more attention to lifting a five-pound weight over his head—a weightlifter or a five-year-old child? The child strains with all his might, and activates a lot of muscles in his back, arms, shoulders, even his legs, some of which aren't even helpful. The weightlifter activates a large yet efficient set of muscles in his arms. And it appears as though our brains are even more efficient and sophisticated than our muscles. After all, the human brain is probably the most complex and evolutionarily adaptive biological mechanism in all of nature."

I had always had a particular fondness for the Venus's flytrap, but

I understood his point. I had grown weary, and felt like I needed to go putt for a while, or have a beer, maybe both. I smiled at him and said softly, "There's a lot here for me to think about." Thinking that I could not possibly pour more information into my own network of neurons, I looked for a way to thank him for his time and end the conversation. Sensing this, he reminded me not to forget to take the pictures of my brain home to my wife and kids. He gave me a large piece of radiologic plastic, with about ten pictures of my brain at different levels of depth, as if it had been sliced into ten sections going from front to back. He joked that I had very large hippocampi on both sides, and said that that was a good thing: "You must have a good memory." As he said this, I recalled his offhand reference to the *self* in the brain. "By the way, what did you mean about the *self* in the brain? How can we understand where the *self* is in the brain?"

He was preparing his things to leave, and was looking down at a pile of papers, not really paying full attention to my question. Then he looked up and stared at me, seeming to look through me as if I weren't there. After a long pause, he said, "People always get confused when I talk about this, but there really isn't a *self* as we think of one. Our experience of self is just the experience of networks connecting with one another. Some people find this depressing, which I don't quite understand. They want to believe that what they feel and experience is how things are, but we can only understand the world by the information that comes to us. We can't see a pure reality; there is only the reality that comes through our senses and into our brains. The more our experiences can be connected to one another through our neuronal networks, the more whole and centered we feel. The feeling of centeredness is determined by how extensive we allow our brain connections to be. You know how people talk in golf about *trusting the shot*? Well, what I'm talking about here is really the basic neuroanatomic underpinnings of trust in ourselves, maybe even the neural circuitry of our faith."

Suddenly, my head didn't hurt anymore. Like at no other time in our conversation, I wanted to hear more from him. Yet he had now gathered his papers and appeared to be in a hurry to leave. "Do you know this feeling of centeredness and faith?" I asked, realizing that all of a sudden I was asking a very personal question.

"Not nearly enough," he said as he smiled and walked away. Then, a ways down the hall, he turned to call out to me, "But I'm working on it all the time!"

~

FOLLOWING OUR INITIAL CONVERSATION, I visited Roland Perlmutter many times to enhance my understanding of the brain and how it works. The meetings were punctuated with his enthusiasm and his hunger for elucidating the mechanisms of brain function. He possessed the type of fascination with the subject of his work I've seen in all of the top scientists I have met. He reminded me of the descriptions I've read about Edison—always tinkering with the model he holds in his mind about how the subject of his interest operates; never deterred, never hopeless, like a sculptor slowly creating a form never before seen by humanity.

Roland's later work, and the work of others in this area over the past few years, will be discussed in the chapters that follow. Roland's initial emphasis on the ventromedial cortex requires slight revision: This region is probably more involved in the unconscious inhibition of incorrect responses and a gathering sense of danger. It is associated more with feeling a negative hunch. This area is crucial for navigating the world and developing trust in oneself, but the ability to follow a positive hunch probably involves inhibiting this region along with activations of areas such as the *caudal anterior cingulate*, which may help us stick to our plans when there is no feedback from the environment telling us we should change.

Before examining this area of research and applying it to how the brain is developed from birth, I first want to move on to the question that I was left with when I first met Roland: How did he work on his own brain function? What did this brain doctor do to make his brain better, to have his neurons migrate to just the right positions so that he could have the experiences and abilities he desired? More important, what techniques were available to all of us to enhance this process? Could athletes learn to shut down the frontal cortex on demand and let their athletic activity originate spontaneously out of them? If so, is this similar to the actions of those who devote their lives to developing centeredness and faith? My conversation with Roland Perlmutter led me to pursue questions that I never even knew existed.

CHAPTER FOUR

Present Perfect

Happiness he who seeks may win, if he practice.

—BUDDHA

The answer is in the dirt.

—HOGAN

W<small>E OFTEN THINK</small> of attention as a spotlight. Our usual impression is that we attend to the objects that are under the direct scrutiny of the light. However, more careful consideration suggests that attention is more like the pattern of waves out at sea; although some of the peaks are sharp and sudden, many roll through our awareness, gradually building importance until we comprehend them, then fading quickly, though not abruptly, through time and memory. You look at the book, then you look up; as you return to the book, even though you're reading attentively, the image of your glance away from the book lingers on, maintained in what is called *working* memory, before it is transferred to long-term memory stores, or fades into neural oblivion. In this manner, what you have thought the moment before affects the thoughts you are having now, which affect the thoughts that are mounting for the future.

We talk about thinking in a way that suggests our thoughts are not experienced as discrete units, but as a continuous stream. *Current* means "happening now," as well as "the part of a fluid body moving continuously in a certain direction." Our attention to what is happening now is experienced as a flowing entity, as a stream of thought that has motion, and that requires movement for us to enter into it. The various meanings of the word *present* also express the ways in which we experience attention: *Present* refers to now, but also to a gift, as well as to the act of bringing something before another. All three of these meanings derive from the fact that the attention of the receiver is focused on the immediate event. When you present me with a gift, I am paying attention to you. I am here at this time. I am present. Yet the converse is also true: When I fully attend to the moment before me, it is presented to me. It is a gift.

Attention to any one thing comes at a cost of attention to other things. Research on cognitive processes has clearly demonstrated that people make choices about the features of the outside world on which they will focus, and these choices determine what information they will collect. A person who is rewarded for paying attention to the colors of briefly flashed stimuli will later not know as much about the location of the stimuli; if the person's strategy is switched to focus on location, her knowledge of color will suffer.

Many great athletes have attributed their successes, and failures, to their powers of concentration. While the psychologist William James assumed that genius led to great powers of attention, it would seem that the converse could also be true: Superior attention enables people to focus more on their skill, digging deeper, refining, honing the art that is the object of their desire. Tiger Woods, the son of a Buddhist mother and soldier father, displays a dramatic ability to focus on the business of the moment. His mother taught him to meditate, and his father recognized his natural ability to focus, then stretched it by teaching him to ignore distractions such as a clap (although apparently not a camera click) in his backswing. Ben Hogan was known to be completely oblivious to aspects of the external world during a tournament round. Rod Laver and John McEnroe reported that, for them, performance was determined by the level of their concentration.

Research studies support the idea that the best athletes in any field often possess the best attentive skills. For instance, novice pistol shooters were found to be *better* at a dual task of responding to a sound with a manual response while preparing to shoot. For the experts, however, as their focus on the primary task of shooting narrowed, the secondary task was relegated to such low status that at times it was ignored. Like Woods and Hogan, they were able to clear the mechanism to narrow their attention as the moment of action approached. Is this because, as James would argue, their genius was so complex that the contents of their mind would catch anyone's attention? Or did the facility of their attention allow their genius to prosper?

Recent research demonstrates that emotion may play a role in narrowing attention even further. When the importance of an event increases, the amount of information that can be absorbed lessens. Some athletes are able to utilize this process to their advantage, while others become crippled by it. Since pressure and, frequently, anxiety result in attention becoming more narrow and internal, an athlete may fail to broaden her attention externally when the situation calls for it. In the closing seconds of a close game, a very nervous point guard may only be able to carry out her coach's diagrammed play, missing her teammate wide open under the basket. A psyched-up quarterback with narrowed peripheral vision may be so focused on one receiver that he cannot see another streaking alone toward the end zone. The trick is to pay attention to what matters, and ignore what doesn't matter. Unfortunately, few athletes and coaches understand that the development of this attention takes practice.

William James was pessimistic that sustained attention could ever be improved, but a wealth of research studies have suggested that he was wrong. Neuroscientists, such as Michael Posner, have described the stages of attention that can be achieved with practice. The first is the *cognitive state*, during which we figure out how to do something, like swing a golf club. The next is the *associative stage*, during which we engrain the act through practice, and develop mental associations between the complex activity and simpler thoughts. The notion of a swing thought is based upon this type of practice. We have dozens of things to think about in the golf swing, but consolidating our mental plans into a single thought is much more efficient, reduces the mental energy devoted to planning, and lets us *do*. Last is the *autonomous stage*, during which our activity becomes less directly subject to cognitive control. Since the motor activity is automatic, it becomes less subject to interference from other ongoing activities or distracting influences. We are at our best when what we are thinking converges with what we are doing. Not that we think about *what* we are doing—the thinking and the doing are the same.

The practice of meditation improves our ability to pay attention to the relevant aspects of our world and allow our thinking and doing to converge. While some of this improvement is not very well understood by scientists, such as how intuition is developed, other components are clear. If we practice interrupting the drifting of our thought processes away from the subject of our attention, such as our breath, we develop an increased ability to control our focus. In this manner, we enlarge the size of the rolling wave of attention that can be devoted to the work in front of us. The relevance to sport performance should be fairly obvious: If a golfer becomes nervous that he is closing in on the best round of his life, and wants to focus on the current shot instead of his intense desire for a low number, the ability to maintain control of his thinking at this crucial time will greatly improve his chances of avoiding the distractions of his expectations. As will be discussed in the next chapter, the purpose of a preshot routine is to hone attention to the relevant aspects of the task at hand. The golfer who can orient himself to the target, not the hazard, and the basketball player who sees only the rim, not the madness behind the backboard, are exercising a mastery of selective attention that can be greatly aided by meditation.

Our usual perception of a master of a craft is that he or she has a special gift. We see the activity unfurl from them and conclude that they must have some special physical or neural attribute that is unavailable to us. Very few of us have the genes that allowed Kobe Bryant's physique to take form, but to take that as indicating a general pattern is a mistake. Most masters developed their craft from an exquisite involvement in its details. Mozart may have been born with an unusual convergence of the auditory and motor systems in his brain that allowed him not only to develop images of the sounds he wanted to create, but also to express those sounds through an instrument at the ends of his fingers. Yet only through daily involvement in this activity could his art take on the complexity that it achieved. The Buddhist monk develops attentive skills through decades of daily practice. He is sometimes bored and sometimes challenged, but only through the investment of time and energy does the mastery of his craft deepen. It's not through magic that a skill develops to the point that it is experienced as springing forth from one's being, it's only through a strong devotion to repeating that skill and understanding the subtleties of its application and misapplication that it can become automatic.

We all have the ability to focus so clearly on the process of an activity that we become completely at one with the activity, but we rarely create the circumstances to allow this. Most people believe that these experiences are not under our control, or they have attempted to have them and failed, so it's best just to hope for them to happen. This is the difference between praying for things to happen to us versus praying for the strength or the courage to allow these things to happen. We can make them more likely by establishing a context for them to arise. While some of that context comes from practicing one's art or skill repeatedly until the activity is automatic, another, far more often ignored component, is making an openness to these experiences a regular part of daily life. Not only will experiencing the unity of action and actor become more likely because you'll have more opportunities, but it will become engrained in every other aspect of your life, further increasing your awareness of opportunities.

Flow and Other Water Analogies to Attention

THE COMPARISONS of attention to water have been with us since at least the time of Buddha, who in the sixth century B.C. described a wise man as he who has "the words of the Dhamma flow into him: He is clear and peaceful like a lake." Like the river that flows continuously, attention is new each moment, yet always dependent upon the previous moment. Mihaly Csikszentmihalyi has written extensively on a mental state of optimal attention in which "people are so involved in an activity that nothing else seems to matter; the experience itself is so enjoyable that people will do it even at great cost, for the sheer sake of doing it." He described the quest for this mental state as "a battle for the self; it is a struggle for establishing control over attention." Csikszentmihalyi has referred to this mental state as *flow*. The use of this term has helped popularize a series of interesting studies performed by him and his colleagues on the relationship between a mental state of *flow* and happiness. The term continues to be used by scientists and the general public.

Csikszentmihalyi described eight (and later nine) components of flow. Recent research by his colleague Susan Jackson with athletes suggests that two factors appear to be most strongly associated with a higher degree of satisfaction with one's athletic performance: the feeling that an activity is being completed for its own sake, and a proper balance between the external challenge and the skills one has to approach that challenge.

The play of healthy children is a prime example of activity completed for its own sake. We are hardwired to experience enjoyment when we learn an activity; while this feels like a reward, it is also a motivation that leads to future competence. Young animals display this type of activity continuously. Note the purposeless activity of tadpoles: They spring spontaneously, for apparently no reason. They are learning to jump, even before they have legs.

Regarding the balance between challenge and skills, if an activity becomes too easy, people get bored and begin thinking of other things. If an activity is too difficult, frustration and self-consciousness may ensue. Sports are ideal for experiencing flow, since they continually provide us with opportunities to challenge ourselves, even as we improve. In this manner, we can often find the right challenge-skills balance that Csikszentmihalyi describes. As we get more proficient at an athletic activity, we then move to another level of challenge. This type of challenge not only enhances our attention on the task of the moment, it demands it.

Some of the research conducted by this group has identified the mechanisms by which flow can be disrupted. Concert pianists have difficulty playing a piece when they become conscious of the notes they're playing, or try to think about how to play the notes, which thus disrupts the flow of movements coming out of them. The classic example is the ease with which one traverses a one-foot-wide plank on the floor, yet placing the plank over a 1000-foot chasm completely changes the activity: The image of disaster causes the walker to focus on what was otherwise a simple, unconscious task, rendering it difficult if not impossible. As Roland Perlmutter has taught me, an abundance of extraneous brain activity occurs when we look at what we're doing instead of just doing it.

Susan Jackson has noted the importance of distinguishing

between self-consciousness and self-awareness. The former is looking at oneself from the outside, which disrupts the feeling of flow. The latter enhances the flow state, as the athlete is attuned to the body and its machinations so that performance can be adjusted whenever the circumstances dictate. However, some of Jackson's recent research indicates that negative feedback about performance leads to more errors, so the self-aware athlete may need to ignore some (negative) aspects of performance in order to maintain a focus on the brilliance that emanates before her. Controlling attention in a manner that facilitates what Csikszentmihalyi calls flow is very difficult, as doing so is self-conscious and, thus, inherently flow disrupting. Buddhist texts describe this dilemma with the saying "once you aim at the target, you have already missed." However, as I have mentioned above, it is possible for the athlete to remove the obstacles for the experience of flow and surround herself with conditions that facilitate it. The book *Flow in Sports*, by Jackson and Csikszentmihalyi, aims to teach athletes how to remove those obstacles, and does a very nice job of it.

The Fertile Ground

About 10,000 years before psychologists began studying attention in the laboratory, the ice of the most recent Ice Age melted away from the land mass now known as Scotland. Its retreat exposed geological faults like the Great Glen, as well as the mossy surface of the basin of the Forth. These east-to-west obstructions served as a barrier between human societies from an uncertain prehistoric time until the end of the first millennium. The result was the development of a relatively isolated culture of people who would eventually call themselves *Scots*, and who would take pride in their differentiation from those in the more southern climes. As Pope Pius II stated in 1435, "nothing gives the Scots more pleasure than to hear the English dispraised."

After the ice was gone, the coast line between the Firths of Tay and Forth fluctuated for about 4,000 years. At times, the seas rose to twenty-five feet above their current level, yet at about 4000 B.C. they made their final retreat, exposing the sandy stretches—the *links*—that centuries of marine transgressions had formed. The stone tools, scrapers, and awls that have been found in these areas indicate that over the next two thousand years men came and went in groups of three or four, perhaps as many as three foursomes, foreshadowing twenty-first-century tourism by staying a week or two at a time in these fauna-rich areas in order to hunt and fish.

The diocese of St. Andrews, which lay in this region between the Firths of Tay and Forth, was one of ten in Scotland in 1155, and perhaps the most important. It was structured similarly to the ancient Celtic monastic churches, owning large endowments of widely scattered land. The kings of this time requested that the pope establish St. Andrews as the metropolitan church of their realm; the largest building in Scotland at the time was the cathedral at St. Andrews. Within the next century, St. Andrews was given honorary royal burgh status by the crown. King David I granted the canons of St. Andrews freedom from tolls in burghs and leave to buy corn and flour for their needs whenever they wished. In addition, the local tradesmen were given freedom from other royal constraints of trade and commerce. St. Andrews was not only a center of religion and commerce, but later, of education, as the first Scottish University was established there in 1411. Even more than the national economic growth of the time, the local economy was well and the local culture was becoming richer.

The common man in this region did not have the resources or idleness of spirit to risk injury or death by engaging in the jousting tournaments of the aristocracy, which required trained horses, expensive weapons and body armor. He was not even rich enough to hunt red deer for sport with hound, bow, and arrow. However, he had time to be safely at leisure with himself. How would this time be filled?

The written history of this time is devoted primarily to the battles of kings and those who would topple them. However, there is evidence that, at about this time, down along the links between the sea and the town of St. Andrews, sheep—the first greenkeepers—grazed on the local grasses, making them short enough for a rock or ball to roll along them, and avoided the wind by sleeping in depressions that would form bunkers. Long before John Hamilton, Bishop of St. Andrews, declared in 1552 that the links of the town be available for townspeople for "golfe, futball, shuting, and all games," and even before the Scottish Parliament under King James II in 1457 decreed that "ye futbawe and ye golf be utterly cryt done and not usyt," golf was born.

It appears as though the game of golf developed in the lap of relative luxury. Only with time idle and safe could such a playful focus on the present emerge. The desperate years were behind the people here, and these were times in which pure experience was celebrated. Unlike work, war, eating, or sex, there was no ulterior purpose to this activity; it was done solely for the experience. The church and the crown disapproved of golf, as it distracted people from the more important activities of attending services to protect their souls against evil, and practicing archery to protect their country against foreigners. The great wars between England and Scotland persisted from 1296 to 1424, and the need for military practice far outweighed the need for a game with ball and club.

Yet golf survived. Golf may have become a respite from violence or even an act of defiance against unwanted authority. Our view of the past is not clear on this point, but time has told us that the genie had escaped from the bottle of human development. Perhaps it had happened during another era, but never before as strong or eventually as far reaching. This development, as simple as it seems, was a billion years in the making: Life on earth had learned to choose to find purpose in the pure moment before it.

Our lives are so luxurious these days that most of us would make the kings of the thirteenth century wild with jealousy, yet we still work very hard. We have developed an enormous bundle of machines to help us with our daily needs, but our needs seem to expand faster than technology can meet them. Each new machine costs us more, so even a healthy economy cannot satisfy us. No matter how much we have, we want more. The moments of focus, of play, have dwindled. No one decides to eliminate them; we just don't put them at the top of our list of things to do. Time and tranquility have again become luxuries. We have returned to the frenetic pace of an age we longed to escape, driven by the promise of the pleasures and bangles of today's marketplace. We have created a war with our world in our attempts to taste its essence. Is there a way to move beyond this seemingly endless cycle?

Roland Perlmutter told me that he worked on this every day through meditation.

Meditation

THERE ARE NUMEROUS FORMS of meditation. Most of them spring from Hindu and Buddhist religious practice. The ancient masters of Hindu yoga defined meditation as the suppression of the movements or operations of the mind. Buddhist forms of meditation generally involve concentrating thought upon a single object, and can be classified into two basic categories: those that act on the mind to induce intuition, and those that settle or still the mind's normal agitation.

It is important to understand that meditating is not a strange or foreign activity. It is not fancy or complicated, but straightforward and simple. Many Western books describe it with Indian or Tibetan terms in italics, making the practice of meditation and the mental states that result from it seem elusive, ethereal. This tendency may enhance readers' attention or perhaps their desire to get away from themselves, but this is an inaccurate reflection of what meditation is and has always been. In the Eastern cultures from which meditation originated, it is a normal, everyday activity. (The parents of an athlete from India once pleaded with me to get their child to eat better and meditate regularly.) Chogyam Trungpa, who developed an organization for teaching Tibetan Buddhist meditation in the United States, Canada, and Europe, deemphasized the mysterious aspects of meditation by referring to it as "sitting." I sit; you sit; so, go sit.

Meditation serves to allow the meditator to access new states of mind that, in theory, are deeper and truer than our normal everyday consciousness. The progression to these conceptually higher, more desired states of mind is usually achieved over the course of years of mediation practice, although any single meditation session can alter the course of a person's mental development. According to Alexandra David-Neel in her classic description of Buddhist tradition, Buddhist meditation that involves the development of reason and intuition directs those who practice it to reject covetousness, anger, indifference, agitation, and doubt. After this, progression continues until reasoning and reflection are also rejected, yet enthusiasm and joy are retained, which allows inner peace and singlemindedness. After enthusiasm has been eliminated, a purer feeling of joy is obtained. Finally, when the meditator has learned to move beyond joy as well as pleasure and suffering, he enters into a neutral state of pure serenity. A PGA Tour player once described to me his approach to putting along the same lines: "I am neutral; I release myself from desire and proceed with the business before me."

When attention is excited, it is almost impossible to keep the mind focused on a single object; your thoughts wander and jump through a forest of ideas, feelings, hopes, and anxieties. When attention becomes lax, it motionlessly settles upon an object, losing clarity and becoming lifeless and dull, leading to lethargy, drowsiness, and, eventually, sleep. By repeatedly recognizing laxity and excitation through introspection, and redirecting attention toward the single object of choice, meditation can aid in the development of mindfulness. The form of meditation that I will focus on here does not involve an abnegation of the self; it is a form of *concentration* that is developed not through conscious strain, but through an enhanced understanding of and appreciation for the moment.

Discipline and routine are important components of meditation. The meditator is instructed to retire to the same room or isolated space where he can be free from external distractions. By utilizing the same space at the same time each day, memories of his previous mental progress enable him through associations to delve into his concentrated state more easily; when the external world is constant and predictable, the meditator can focus his attention on the complexity of the mind before him. The preparation to meditate often elicits an experience of evening, which is explained in Buddhism through a simile of the sea, in which the reflection of the world, normally rippled by the agitation of the mind, becomes as smooth as a mirror.

When one meditates, ideas rise into awareness with great frequency and rapidity, each one flitting about before being replaced by the next. Meditation practice aims to gain control of thought processes through introspection, which enables the meditator to recognize and inhibit the constant stream of thought, allowing mindfulness. Buddhist text describes that following meditation, "the condition which one has then obtained resembles that of a man who, from the river bank, watches the water flow past. Even so the mind, observant and calm, watches the passing of the uninterrupted flux of ideas which hurry after one another."

Roland Perlmutter introduced me to the form of meditation that he had practiced for almost thirty years. It originated in Tibet, and is very straightforward. He said it helped him enter into the state of consciousness that he called the *effortless present:* "the frame of mind in which nothing seems to exist other than the vivid explosion of the moment. All actions seem to spring out of you on their own." To practice it, you simply sit in a place where interference from the external world can be minimized, and allow yourself to become one with the exhale of your breath. Face straight ahead, with your gaze softly fixed upon a point on the ground in front of you. Buddhist texts describe that the spine should be "as straight as a stack of coins," but some Western bodies will have trouble with this posture, and one should avoid becoming rigid or uncomfortable. When your mind drifts to other topics, like the many things you have to do today, your anxieties about the future, your relationships, and your sexual fantasies, you simply, silently, label the stream of thoughts as *thinking*, then return your focus to your oneness with your exhale. This interrupts the constant chattering of your mind that fills the spaces in your usual perception of and interaction with the outside world. This practice helps you to realize the many thoughts that come and go in a brief period of time. You see that in the past, when someone has asked you what you were thinking, and you said "nothing," that this is almost impossible. Thinking continues on like radio waves from a tower, relentlessly beaming energy to the center of your attention.

It is important not to be critical of the fact that your attention regularly and repetitively abandons its focus on the exhale, and devolves into thinking. Even describing this wandering as *devolving* is judgmental; merely label it as *thinking*, then shift your attention to your breath again. Many people give themselves a hard time about this: "I can't believe that I can't keep my attention on my breath!" However, this level of arousal only solidifies your attention away from your exhale and expresses the degree of difficulty that you, like most of us, have in controlling your thought processes. Such is the rhythm of the meditating mind: toward focus, away from focus, straining to focus, now agitated that focus is not where it is intended to be, back to focus. Meditation enables the mind to bring itself back to the activity of the moment, which in this practice is the breath.

This is also the rhythm of the properly tuned mind in athletics. The constant chatter in the background of many athletes' minds is usually directed toward the context and importance of the athlete's activity: "How am I playing?" "What does coach think?" "I wonder what the cut is going to be today?" "I'm four under. Can I really keep playing this well?" The trained mind of an athlete interrupts this flow of thought with attention to the current moment. She has developed an ability to replace the monitoring process with a more serene, accepting mental stance. Many research studies have found that decreasing self-criticism in the midst of competition greatly improves performance. When you allow your breath to be expelled from your lungs, when the natural and cyclical flow of air between your body and the outside world can be observed unimpeded, then you begin to gain control over your tendency to intervene when intervention is unnecessary. You begin to let unfold what is harmonic in you and between you and the rest of the world. You return from the agitated mental state of internal chattering to a direct focus on the activity in front of you. In this mental state, which Roland called the *effortless present*, athletic activity is experienced as springing effortlessly to life in front of the athlete.

As a stillness of mind is developed through meditation, another, more complex, transformation occurs. From the sanctuary of our observation post, we see that much of our knowledge is based upon our individual biases. If something causes us pleasure, we struggle to increase our knowledge of it; if something causes us pain, we struggle to ignore it. As we observe this bias, we nurture the growth of another type of awareness, a discriminating awareness that doesn't evaluate or judge the worth of something to us, one that sees things as they are without our personal bias. We begin to appreciate the difference between what we know based upon our own particular histories, and what we know because it's true.

In Buddhist teaching, attention to daily activities is enhanced through the same process as the practice of meditation. When engaged in an activity, such as walking to the store, the mind drifts toward similar subjects that may confront the meditator. These are also labeled as *thinking*, though the shift of attention is not toward the breath, but toward the activity in which one is engaged. The walker may see a car that reminds her of an old boyfriend, which makes her remember a pleasant romantic moment, leading to a consideration of her current relationship; this is then labeled as *thinking*, and the attention is returned toward walking. She feels her foot on the pavement, which receives the heel and aids the transfer of energy to the toe before beginning again. The breeze softly swirls her hair, and single strands brush her cheek. She is walking. She feels the beginning of each step and the ending of the other simultaneously, in rhythm, as the separate instruments of a band playing their part of the same song. Another car passes by, perhaps another associative memory. Birds fly overhead. She feels lifted. She labels her thinking and is back to a focus on walking. These shifts in attention may not be easy to accomplish. She may forget to label her thinking. She may decide that one of the memories she is having is more pleasurable than her attention to the present. Yet her persistence will discipline her mind to focus on her task at hand, regardless of what it is.

Meditation tends to facilitate later attempts to return to the present activity. First, memories of having meditated earlier that day, or even the night before, will remind us to label our mental wanderings as *thinking* and return to the present. As we spend more time in a meditative state, it influences how we think of ourselves, which then infiltrates the later moments in our lives. In this manner, meditation serves the rather mundane role of a refrigerator magnet, reminding us of what we want to be and how we want to live. The work of our previous meditation also serves to keep fresh the feelings we had while meditating. Our emotional memory of the meditative session thus becomes easier to access later in the day, smoothing our way to revisit the same level of attention to our everyday activity. We recall the grace that the meditative moment created, and we are inspired and encouraged to let this happen again, resonating through the day.

If we can learn to attend to the repetitive, monotonous, and boring flow of our breath, then giving our attention to athletic activity such as a six-foot putt for par or a free throw becomes relatively easy. These athletic events are so much better able to capture our interest. If we solidify the process of returning our attention to simple and commonplace activities, such as our breath or our walking, we can then apply this process to the complexity of athletic activities. The psychological exercise of recognizing thinking and shifting focus toward oneness with the breath nurtures unbiased, observing attention in the isolated chamber of meditation. The breath comes and goes regardless of our effort. We experience the breath without needing to do anything and, when we wander away, it is there awaiting our return. In this stable context we can best learn how our mind wanders. The breath is also the role model for our serenity: unwavering, cyclical, dependable, alive in the present. When the meditator emerges from meditation practice, he is better able to control how he attends to the world of his everyday life.

Since our breath rarely requires effort, paying attention to it is more of an exercise than attending to our athletic activities. Drawing back a putter or releasing a basketball toward the rim usually requires our attention to the activity. However, our desire for an outcome makes the mental approach to our putt or shot more complicated. We can assume that we will breathe successfully if we need to do that; the destiny of our putt is not as certain. Athletic activity is a more interesting object of our attention, but it is also more influenced by our wish for a particular future. We want a specific result, and lose our perspective as observer, thrusting our consciousness from the present to the uncertainty of the future. Meditative practice can completely transform the normal approach to these athletic moments. By learning to approach the initiation of athletic activity in the same zealless manner that the meditator greets his breath, the athlete can let go of his desire to alter the future and allow the present to be fully and vigorously expressed.

~

INSTEAD OF FEELING BLISSFUL, relaxed, and immediately rewarded, I've found meditation a challenge. I sometimes feel alternately self-conscious, restless, and sleepy while meditating; I usually want to get up and leave. I'm very happy when I don't; there often comes a time when there is a presentation of a peaceful few seconds, and I have the thought that "this is right." Sometimes I follow this present-state focus with a future-oriented pledge to "do this more." My attention is usually different immediately after I've meditated; I am more aware of my immediate environment, and I feel less need to act on my impulses and anxieties. My perceptions are slightly more vivid, but only if I attend to them. Sometimes, I remember my postmeditation state of mind later in the day, and I can remind myself to slide back into this open, waiting, mindful consciousness. This type of mental state lets me consciously focus on the current moment. It's as though my intentions are resolved by releasing them and allowing them to come to life in the effortless present. These moments are very similar to the experience I had of the club swinging itself years ago.

I've found in my sport psychology practice that many athletes won't meditate, even if they're told to do so. It seems weird and foreign to them, and can alienate them from me in our work together. Further, while the accouterments of meditation, that is, sitting in the lotus position or burning incense, facilitate meditative consciousness for some people, to others they're distracting. So, instead of using the word *meditate*, I emphasize that they are working on their focus and concentration, whether by sitting and breathing or by focusing on their everyday activities. Many athletes, just like the meditators, try to motivate themselves to do a better job at this activity, and berate themselves for not focusing on the task. One football player told me that the wandering away from his mind would initially be labeled as *thinking*, but, after he had drifted away a few times, his thinking would transform into "Come on, moron, you're thinking again, concentrate on brushing your —ing teeth!" Just as in actual meditation practice, this self-criticism is informative, because it shows the athletes how they treat themselves even when they're given a benign task, but it doesn't facilitate the meditative state. They need to learn to approach the wandering of their attention in a less judgmental way. I teach them to acknowledge that the mind has drifted, label the *thinking*, and return to the task at hand. These exercises improve their focus and teach them to treat their consciousness more gently, which produces associations between the concentration exercise and affirmation.

I serendipitously stumbled onto an easy exercise that facilitates a meditative state of mind before practicing golf. I had taken a few golf lessons from Ed Ibarguen, a PGA Master Professional and general manager of the Duke University Golf Club. He taught me to work on my alignment with a three-foot piece of vinyl cord tied to golf tees at each end. The tees are placed in the ground, and the cord creates a perfectly straight line to develop an aligned setup. The cord is very light and, when wrapped around the tees, it's no larger than the inner core of a wound golf ball. Like much of Ed's advice, it has been tremendously useful, and I frequently recommend it to others, since the usual procedure of laying down clubs can make golfers feel confined. Further, if a golfer fears hitting the clubs on the downswing, the practice can encourage a swing path that is too much down the line.

One of the drawbacks of the cord, however, is that if it's left in one's golf bag for an extended period of travel or play, it often becomes a mass of knots. After the repeated frustration of having to disentangle knots for five minutes before hitting balls, I wanted to go back to using clubs for alignment practice. I became especially frustrated when I was in a hurry, or very eager to practice. Then I realized that the challenge of slowing down my fevered mental pace, so that I could focus on untangling the cord, was the exact proper prelude to hitting balls. Working with the knots requires patient attention so as not to increase their tightness, yet the knots are often so complex it's almost impossible to develop a real strategy for untying them. Getting a feel for the task demands persistent, gentle tugging, allowing the knots to become untied, and the feedback between the cord and the fingers seems almost to bypass the brain. The task is inherently calming, since it can only be accomplished by being calm. Whenever I use the cord now, by the time the knot is untied, my mind is much calmer and focused, and I'm ready to take a similar approach to my practice. It enhances my view of golf not as a series of knotty problems that should have been solved already, but as an endless string of opportunities to create solutions.

~

LONG BEFORE THE TERM *karma* was bastardized by Western rock-star gurus and their followers, it referred to the cause and effect of volitional action. The notion is that if you go about your life grasping tightly to the control of your intentions, making only deliberate decisions and effortful acts, your world will be limited to these actions and the reaction of the outside world to them. Meditation serves to move a person beyond this chain-reaction world of controlled acts and their effects. Movement would then be experienced as coming not from an individual's personal and selfish concerns, but rather from a universal state of higher awareness. Many writers and philosophers have suggested that this control of attention and its resultant egoless mental state begets great intelligence. William James stated in 1890 that "the faculty of voluntarily bringing back a wandering attention, over and over again, is the very root of judgment, character, and will. . . . An education which should improve this faculty would be *the* education *par excellence.*"

In chapter 2, I introduced the idea that some coincidences may be due to unconscious, sometimes shared, knowledge. Chapter 3 described some of the possible brain mechanisms involved in the development of this awareness. While this perspective seems to take the fun out of synchronous experiences, its implications are bigger than coincidences and magical concepts like mind reading. It points to the fact that we have the ability to be much smarter than we recognize. We know far more than we allow ourselves to realize, and we are able to act on information that we do not know we have. Allowing ourselves access to this intelligence creates enormous possibilities for our personal power. Meditation and prayer appear to increase our ability to access this type of attention. If this is so, then why doesn't everyone make these meditative exercises a part of every day? Perhaps we limit ourselves, as Nelson Mandela once said, because we are afraid of how powerful we really are. An Indian philosopher named Krishnamurti said that, if the whole human race were taught to cultivate this intelligence, many of the world's problems would be solved. I am not sure I understand what he meant by this, or how it would work, but it seems right to me somehow.

When we adopt this approach to our lives, each moment is a perfect opportunity to be present. Our tennis is a game of moments unfolding in rhythmic bliss, our work is enjoyable, and our golf *is* a game of perfect. Solidly struck, with our finish position balanced and quietly confident, the ball bounds down the green fairway, pulled by gravity, pushed by force, slowed by friction, and rests in a depression filled with sand polished by rushing water and relentless time. An opportunity to rise to the challenge of the fairway bunker awaits. This is not perfect?

CHAPTER FIVE

Sport Psychology Consultation
(The Introject on Your Shoulder)

This is a lonely, lonely life; sorrow is everywhere you turn . . . and that is worth some money if you think about it, that is worth some money.

— SINGER-SONGWRITER PAUL SIMON
DISCUSSING SPORT PSYCHOLOGISTS ON THE
PGA TOUR IN "RHYTHM OF THE SAINTS"

M Y EXPERIENCE OF THE CLUB moving on its own that day in New Jersey had raised all kinds of questions for me about the nature of human movement, how it can be facilitated by exercises like meditation, and how it's regulated by the brain. It also inspired me to shift the focus of my career. I began to feel, as do most people who become even mildly taken with golf, that the mental side is the weakest part of anyone's game, and it can benefit from instruction even more than the physical parts of the game. Since the time of my training in clinical psychology, I had heard of sport psychology, but I had no idea how this field really worked. I read a few books on how to improve the mental side of one's golf, and thought that the techniques were interesting and effective. Many of these techniques were essentially practical ways to help athletes enter into what Roland Perlmutter described as the effortless present. I began to consider changing my career from neuroscience researcher and clinical psychologist to sport psychologist. When Dick Coop, who does sport psychology consultation for several prominent PGA Tour players and college athletes at UNC–Chapel Hill, agreed to train me in the techniques of sport psychology, I jumped at the chance. I found a position as a researcher down the street at Duke, where I could work while training with Dick. My initial consultations were with golfers whom Dick sent me, but eventually my practice grew to include other sports.

Sport psychology is a funny field. The FDA requires that, before a new medication can be approved for use, the manufacturer must demonstrate that it is effective and its side effects are minimal. There is no such regulation of sport psychology techniques. The field is in its infancy, and there hasn't been enough time for research to address the efficacy or potential psychological side effects of these techniques. How does a professional golfer distinguish an experienced teacher of the mental game from a quack? Sometimes, not very well. While no one would argue that someone having had seventeen heart surgeries qualifies him to perform surgery on others, some people seem to think their psychological life experience is qualification enough for them to help others in the psychological aspect of their sport. One professional golfer I knew said that he would never take lessons from anyone who had not won a major championship; Lee Trevino used to say that he'd never take advice from anyone who could not beat him. A sport psychologist friend of mine told me that, when he was in graduate school, the women's basketball coach at his university would not give his ideas much attention because she was receiving counsel from a local used-car dealer who referred to himself as a "sports psychologist" even though he had no formal training. It's hard to say why she preferred the car dealer to the graduate student, but apparently she was getting something that she needed—although there's an equal possibility that she was getting a lemon and didn't know the difference.

Sport psychology societies have tried to restrict the use of the term *sport psychologist* to those who have a Ph.D. in sport psychology. This means that people like me and Dr. Coop, who have received doctoral training in fields such as counseling college students or doing psychotherapy, cannot call themselves sport psychologists, which is probably for the best (I don't, and neither does Dr. Coop). However, the most severe punishment for this unethical behavior is to be asked to leave societies such as the American Psychological Association; the used-car dealers don't belong to these societies, so they can call themselves whatever they want. In the end, it comes down to whether the athlete can trust someone enough to open up his internal world.

Every year, in his talk to PGA Tour rookies, Dick Coop asks them whether they use a swing teacher and a sport psychologist. The number using a sport psychologist has grown to the point that more Tour players use one than use a swing teacher. Perhaps the best individual endorsement in history for sport psychology is the fact that, since he was thirteen, Tiger Woods has spent time with a sport psychologist, who also frequently caddied for Tiger in important amateur tournaments.

Why do so many Tour players use sport psychologists? I think one of the main reasons is that golfers, especially professional golfers, need to tell their story to someone. Most of the people in the lives of serious golfers are too personally involved with them or their game to be a receptive and objective ear, or are ignorant of the complexities of the game, or are just not interested enough to listen to the details of each round. (Tour caddie joke, while Tour player starts to describe his entire round, shot by shot: "Are we going eighteen? 'Cause if we are, I'd like to take a cart.")

The sport psychologist not only gets paid to listen to whatever the golfer wants to talk about, but he or she actually considers these details to be an important part of the working relationship. Further, he or she may ask additional questions about the round and how the golfer was feeling and thinking before and after some shots. In this manner, the golfer and the psychologist create a narrative of the golfer's inner life. It's not something that anyone can easily do alone; some of the subtle emotions that an athlete experiences during the course of his or her sport cannot be accessed without a considerable amount of verbal expression. As the golfer remembers and expresses these thoughts and emotions to the psychologist—who, presumably, is listening and understanding—a connection develops between them that is unlike any other.

One of the unspoken yet essential components of a successful sport psychology consultation is that, as the golfer continues to open up about his experiences on the golf course, he'll begin to refer to the psychologist in his mind while he is playing, and be comforted by this image of someone who wants him to succeed, grow, and develop. If the psychologist can provide a nurturing and accepting environment, the golfer will recall images of previous benevolent relationships, allowing him to feel further buoyed by the relationship with the psychologist. The development of this type of relationship was initially described in detail by Freud, who referred to it as *transference*. This view is largely unpopular with most sport psychologists, since it not only seems to minimize what they do ("he's only playing better because he feels as though you want him to"), but also because it places their work in the realm of psychotherapy, where interpersonal dynamics, especially those between shrink and shrinkee, become the focus of attention. Sport psychologists receive minimal training in this aspect of human interaction, so they often ignore it. Avoiding this issue may hamper the ability of the psychologist to address fundamental questions, such as what drives the athlete to participate and excel, yet it probably has little effect on the ability of the psychologist to help the athlete enhance his or her performance.

Golf is a very lonely game, especially when you play it for a living.

The golfer who opens up to someone about his moment-to-moment experiences on the golf course is not as alone; he has an internal image, an *introject*, on his shoulder throughout his round. Anyone who has felt "I can't make it alone" doesn't have to: All it takes is enough money to pay the hourly fee. And, if that's too expensive, there are many used-car dealers who you may feel are just as good.

This may help explain why the increased stress of playing on the PGA Tour has led more players to work with sport psychologists than ever before, and it also may explain why many people do not want to work with one. Some people think sharing one's real internal world with another is a sign of weakness. I have often heard people say, "Ben Hogan wouldn't have used a sport psychologist." I agree. Ben Hogan seemed to have a very strong mental game, and he chose to live a life of fairly consistent isolation from other people. According to some who knew him, Hogan's "secret" may have been a mental image of a supportive compatriot, Hennie Bogan, who eliminated the need for him to rely upon other people. I don't know if that makes Ben Hogan stronger or weaker than modern PGA Tour players.

I believe that, for anyone to be successful in an isolated pursuit like a golf career, they need someone to serve as this introject. In Hogan's time, the majority of sports endeavors were between-war proving grounds for manhood. Expressing complicated emotions about success and failure not only had no place in the arena, but there was a strong tendency to extinguish them internally as well. There was obviously a practical reality to this, since ambivalence on the battlefield leads quickly to death. The vestiges of this mentality are evident throughout sport, although they've retreated considerably. The global battle against terrorism may increase this mentality, if young people again have to prepare for war.

Men and women tend to differ here. I know that generalizing about sex differences puts one on thin ice, and I will skate lightly.

However, the research findings are consistent with my personal experience, so I feel confident that I'm making a relatively objective statement when I say that young women (college age and younger) tend to be more open to sport psychology interventions than young men. This difference may change when a young man tries to work at his sport for a living, but not always. Women are generally more likely to open themselves up to other people when they're having difficulty. Research suggests that when female athletes are stressed, they tend to avoid conflict but express sadness and disappointment. The extreme of this tendency is depression, which affects women three times more often than men. On the other hand, men are more likely to deal with stress by denying the emotional components of it, and by trying to fix the source of the problem, such as thinking about solutions and controlling the stressful situation. This action-oriented approach makes men nine times more likely than women to develop alcoholism. When attempting to solve problems, men and women also tend to differ a bit: Women are more likely to involve other people in their solutions, by obtaining assistance or seeking information. (Note to men: This is why they want to ask for directions when they are lost.) Men may refrain from seeking help when solving problems because of social sanctions against such behavior, and because they're more likely to respond to stress by avoiding social contact. (Note to women: This is one reason why they don't want to ask for directions; the other, as mentioned earlier, is that they like to follow their hearts, and may even want to impress their women with how well they do so.) Research on Olympic athletes suggests that female runners are more likely to react to a slump with greater emotion such as getting angry and seeking sympathy, while male runners are more likely to react to a slump with problem-focused coping strategies.

Some golfers, even professionals, refuse to use sport psychology techniques for fear that they'll be duped into developing beliefs that are untrue. Such a golfer seems to feel as though there is only one real emotion inside him—and, if it's negative, he needs to respect it and leave it alone. If someone has not recovered from disappointment, it is hopelessness that springs eternal: Seeking help from someone else would be a move toward improving expectations, and possibly further disappointment. So, he stands frozen in his isolated individualism, the final lonely holdout in a windswept deserted town.

I had frequent interactions with a professional golfer who felt this way. He had been one of the top junior golfers in the country when he was younger, but his dismal outlook prevented him from finding success in professional tournament golf. I offered numerous times to help him, and he said he would think about it, but he never followed up. During one conversation he said, "I just don't need anyone telling me to think positively." He might as well have said, "No one can connect with my darkness, so don't try; I'm going to hold onto it no matter how much it destroys me!" I tried to challenge him by asking, "Do you want to be right, or do you want to be great?" His silence answered my question. He wound up moving to California to buy a driving range, which failed, and is now an assistant golf pro.

One fascinating tendency in this area is the declaration from a golfer who has just shot repeated stellar rounds that "I don't want to talk about it." I have seen several golfers on minitours respond this way to shooting consecutive scores in the low sixties. In general, I think this forebodes failure: The refusal to acknowledge great success and incorporate it into your being leaves the success compartmentalized and isolated. The golfers who have done this have had none of the overall success that their low scores would suggest is inside them.

At this point, or perhaps long before, you may have found yourself questioning my authority on this subject: "Unless he's been there, how does he know what the athlete is really experiencing?" I'll refrain from the argument of the orthopedist can understand what's wrong with someone's knee without having had knee problems, since that argument is limited to the treatment of pathological conditions, and understanding the psychology of excellence and mastery is different from understanding psychopathology. A better argument is that sport psychologists are essentially mental coaches, and some of the best coaches were mediocre players (a local guy named Krzyzewski comes to mind). However, I think the most important factor is that the brain is organized so that entirely different neural networks govern our actions and our understanding of the mechanisms of those actions. As discussed in chapter 3, the action of athletes is usually associated with activation of the motor cortex; the more automatic and grooved an action is, the less it will coincide with activation in the frontal cortex, the area that observes movements and notices trends, feelings, and errors. Thus, the athlete who is making the most skilled movements, and likely the most automatic movements, is very possibly the person who is least able to observe and report what he or she did.

Joseph Campbell referred to the hero as one with "a thousand faces." In superior athletes, none of those faces is looking within. Athletes frequently give inaccurate reports about internal experiences. High-level tennis players say that they keep their eye on the ball during its entire flight toward them. For decades, there was no reason and no evidence to dispute this sensible claim, yet studies of their eye movements have shown that they look away from the ball at crucial moments as it approaches. In fact, tennis players respond much more to the body movements of their opponents to determine where the ball will be coming than they do to the actual ball flight. So, while it may still be true that "those who can, do; those who can't, teach," those who make the best doers don't necessarily make the best teachers. Internal experience is limited, and while the center of the arena may still be the best place to be, it might not be the best source from which to learn what happens there.

I looked to all of the fundamental techniques of sport psychology to try to understand what had happened to me on the driving range in New Jersey, and also how it could be applied to the inner lives of the athletes I had begun to train. The cornerstone principles of sport psychology include imagery, concentration, relaxation, routines, and self-talk. Many of these techniques help golfers bring their complete focus to the task in front of them, to allow their athletic ability to flow forth effortlessly from them. Since it was a visual image that had had such a profound effect on me on that driving range, I explored imagery first and most extensively.

Imagery

ALTHOUGH LANGUAGE may be what most distinguishes us from other animals, it's our ability to develop images of our intentions that drives us. Motor imagery, commonly referred to as *visualization*, is probably the most fundamental application of sport psychology principles. The term *motor imagery* is probably more accurate, since the images that are used in sport are predominantly *kinesthetic* (how it feels to move) rather than *visual* (what it looks like to move), although most people seem to use both. The idea that an internal image of action can improve the ease and accuracy of that action is now well accepted in sport science and neuroscience. Imagery techniques have been found to be effective in a vast array of athletic and nonathletic movements, from sinking putts to playing oboe to landing the space shuttle. Studies of negative imagery have indicated that performance can also be impaired by images of an incorrect method of completing a motor task, such as golf putting. Other researchers have demonstrated that even tiny and largely meaningless movements, such as pinky strength, can be greatly improved through the use of imagery practice.

Most imagery exercises have greater relevance than pinky-strength development. High-profile athletes have been singing the praises of imagery for the past few decades. On his way to hitting 70 home runs in 1998, Mark McGwire described his routine of imagining the perfect swing and perfect contact; he could be seen in the dugout, eyes closed, while he awaited his turn at bat. Hundreds of major league pitchers have followed the techniques of Steve Carlton, who in the 1970s described his pregame routine of imagining every single pitch he would throw for a nine-inning game. Many football teams get together in their hotel the night before a game, usually meeting by position, to visualize the plays they'll make the next day. While the use of imagery was once considered a cutting-edge technique, it is now commonplace; I recently polled a group of about 150 female high-school lacrosse players prior to a talk on sport psychology, and about half of them had already used imagery techniques.

No sport benefits more from imagery than golf. Ever since Jack Nicklaus was reported to have said that he did not swing the club until he was able to see the shot he wanted to hit, golfers have worked to refine the ability to image the flight of the ball and the swing of the club. Golf magazines are littered weekly with quotes from Tour players describing the effectiveness or ineffectiveness of their images, and the relation of these images to their performance. Despite the attention these techniques have received, I've been surprised by how many golfers use them without really understanding what they're doing.

There are various types of imagery and imagery techniques. The content of the images can vary greatly depending on the purpose a person is trying to serve, from technical refinement to control of emotions. Most people think that all imagery techniques involve seeing oneself performing an activity from a third-person perspective, as in "I can see myself from behind standing over the ball, now getting in the slot at the top of my backswing, through to the perfect finish position." This technique is used very often, and it can be very effective, but many athletes prefer to use imagery from a first-person perspective, both visual and kinesthetic: They imagine what they will see when they engage in an activity, or they imagine what the activity will *feel* like.

The external, third-person view is used most frequently by people beginning a sport, since it lets them see how a complex act is performed, then make plans to perform it. This type of imagery also enables a highly experienced athlete to learn the more complex aspects of a skill, such as a new move in a gymnastics routine. One of the research assistants in my laboratory, who practiced aikido, learned about motor imagery for the first time while helping me design a brain-imaging study of imagery techniques. She began to apply it to her aikido practice, and found that she was much better able to learn a complex new move when she pictured herself doing it several times first. The external view may also be helpful in learning to detect errors in a sequence of complex moves. Beginning golfers can use it to incorporate information about the golf swing; watching a Tour player on television, then imagining oneself swinging the club the same way may not be realistic, but it gets the brain thinking about how the swing should be made.

First-person imagery that focuses on what the athlete will see when involved in the activity is generally most effective for skills that require a response to the external world. Downhill skiers use this technique to practice the points during a race at which they'll begin a turn. One of the Duke quarterbacks found this particularly effective in learning a new offense that was installed before his junior year. The offense required him to see all of the receivers downfield, which had been a weakness of his; he visualized each receiver's pass route individually, and when he had a very clear visual image of that receiver, he would move on to the next. Then, once he felt that he had clear images of each individual receiver, he began to see two, then three in combination, until he could see the whole play develop before him. It is important to note that this imagery was practiced from *his* perspective. He visualized the play developing as he'd see it while dropping back in the pocket to pass. This allowed him to develop a realistic perspective on the play, not just a theoretical view of the play from the press box or end zone, where most game-film cameras are located. He felt it let him see a play develop more fully, and he became better at finding open receivers as a result. This type of technique is useful to coaches when teaching new skills or strategies, like how to recognize and defend against a particular offense in basketball. Some coaches may feel that this benefit is outweighed by the team's reaction when they say, "Okay, now, close your eyes and picture yourself . . ." However, I've seen coaches very effectively bring this type of imagery into their everyday communications with their players in a less formalized way.

The most frequently used imagery technique for the most experienced athletes is to generate images of how an action *feels*. These internal, kinesthetic images may be more helpful than the external perspective in making the skill engrained. A kinesthetic image of doing is the single purest way to prime the motor cortex to move. The image activates the regions associated with the movement, and neural activity prior to the actual movement is as important as getting blood to a muscle by warming it up before testing its strength and flexibility. While this type of imagery can be used at any point in time, even during a brief interlude in a game, such as when a basketball goes out of bounds, it is most useful when the athlete initiates the action and has control of the timing of his movement, such as at the free throw line.

The distinction between the internal and external perspectives may be somewhat artificial. After all, one of the consistent characteristics of the human brain is that it uses whatever information it can to make performance easier and more efficient. Some recent research has shown that imagining one's self from a distance may also activate the motor areas in the brain responsible for this movement. In some studies, the most experienced athletes (e.g., Olympians) reported that when they use external perspectives in their imagery, they experience simultaneous kinesthetic sensations. Recent functional imaging studies have demonstrated that even watching videotapes of someone else doing an action activates the part of a person's own motor cortex that performs the task. Piano players, as opposed to those with no piano experience, will activate the finger-movement regions of the brain even if they are just passively listening to music. Occasionally, people report that watching the movements of others will in fact elicit feelings of the movements in themselves. I remember watching my brother-in-law feed my niece when she was an infant; he was totally unaware that each time he moved the spoonful of food toward her mouth, he opened up his own mouth as well. When I pointed this out to him, he found that he couldn't stop doing it, which became almost ticklish to him, and he burst into laughter whenever it happened.

For athletes, the overlap between the visual and kinesthetic neural systems may help them switch from external to internal imagery. Runners sometimes report that they love to watch the smoothness and rhythm of another runner; that image, whether they're watching it or imagining it, gives them a feeling they want to achieve. I've told runners to imagine that other runner in front of them, graceful, strong, possessing whatever characteristics she wants. Then, as she closes the distance between herself and the other runner, she should feel those characteristics in herself, feel the other's power and fluidity, almost as if she had entered the other's body and the other was *running* her. Over time, she will get the feeling that she has adopted the characteristics of the other runner into her own body, incorporated them into herself.

Imagery can not only help develop and engrain ideal motor performance, but also aid in handling adversity. After a particularly poor shot, many golfers feel overcome with emotion and negative images, as though they'll never hit a good shot again. Repeated images of the ideal swing and ball flight can expunge the havoc wrought by negative images. This is particularly effective if he can call up the images in immediate response to the poor shot, before the memory trace of the poor shot can be imprinted and repeated. As discussed earlier, a lot of research suggests that emotions enhance memory; the vivid slow-motion details that a person may recall after having a car accident is one example. Usually, this works against us on the golf course: We curse our bad shots repeatedly, and play them over in our minds, engraining the negativity to the point that we expect nothing else. However, we can also make this feature of memory work in our favor, interrupting the downward spiral with repeated images of the shot that we *wanted* to hit, followed by enthusiastic emotions about the new, positive images. The next shot will then be imbued with positive expectations instead of looming disaster. This exercise works in other sports as well, such as in basketball when a player feels he's not shooting well on a particular night.

A preround routine of imagining each shot of an upcoming eighteen-hole round can infuse confidence into a golfer, and establish a series of images that can be called upon later, in the midst of the round. Part of this preround routine can include images that help develop and solidify plans to respond to some challenges the golfer may encounter. For instance, many golfers lose strokes by making impulsive decisions to try high-risk shots. Although these shots are appealing at the time, in retrospect the golfer sees that he could have avoided several strokes by following a more conservative plan. Such a plan can be developed, engrained, then carried out on the course through imagery. Before the round, the golfer might envision himself facing the second shot on a par-5 with a green protected by water. He imagines the temptation to hit a driver from the fairway, but then sees himself recalling his plan, laying up, then making birdie anyway. When he gets in this or a similar situation on the course later, he'll be more likely to follow the more conservative plan that will probably save several shots. (I don't necessarily advocate this conservative approach. Golf magazines tell us that a conservative approach will lead to lower scores, which is certainly true; the reason this advice is repeated so often, and so rarely followed, is that, while recreational golfers may want lower scores, they also want to remember hitting great shots. I think that David Toms' decision to lay up on the 72nd hole of the PGA Championship in 2001 was courageous and brilliant, and I would hope that any professional golfer who has worked with me would be able to make the same decision. I, however, would most likely not have done it. Unlike David Toms, I would have probably been about to complete a mediocre round that meant nothing to anyone but me, and the five-wood over the water would have been my last opportunity at glory, so I might indeed have taken the chance.)

During the course of a preround imagery session, a golfer may see himself hitting a poor shot. This is a great opportunity to plan what his response to disappointment on the course will be. As part of the imagery, he can envision beginning to lose control of his emotions, then picture how he will approach the next shot, using his preshot routine to help him completely focus on the present. Such a response to adversity can be solidified and later remembered by including an image of the warm glow of satisfaction for his restraint, and confidence in his temperament.

~

ANOTHER WAY TO USE IMAGERY to fight adversity is in handling fear. All athletes have to deal with fear at some point, and unwanted images of disaster are common. Every sport has its own version of the dream in which one is back in elementary school unclothed, whether it's dropping a pass wide open in the end zone or missing a free throw or a layup as the buzzer goes off. No athletes are completely immune to it. Bobby Jones described that when tapping in a six-inch putt to win the U.S. Open, he became so overcome with the fear that he was about to stub his putter on the ground behind the ball, that he purposely topped the ball into the cup.

Fear in this type of situation usually develops from the negative images that compete with our desires. The typical response to these images is to try to ignore them. Unfortunately, this is no more effective than Dostoyevsky's brother's efforts to not think of a white elephant. The slicer who sees out-of-bound stakes right on a hole, and tries not to think about the possibility of hitting his third (or fifth!) shot from the same tee, is likely doomed. I once worked with a professional golfer who faced a very tricky, downhill, left-to-right, three-foot putt. She hit a weak little push of a putt, and it ambled up to the right of the cup. When I asked her if she was thinking about the *next* putt, she responded that she was trying not to.

Research studies have demonstrated that our feared images sit in our minds like a cartoon bubble hovering above one's head. A technique used in anxiety management called *focus and release* can help control imagery in these situations when fear arises. The feared outcome is confronted directly, including even a full image of the potential disaster. The golfer sees the ball sail out of bounds, sees herself cursing the shot, sees herself hitting three from the tee, annoyed and disheartened. It is important that she not jump away from that image too quickly but, instead, very deliberately push the image aside and visualize the shot that she *is* going to hit. She then proceeds with her preshot routine with the new, fresh image as the beacon guiding her through the darkness.

Imagery can also engrain the expectation of confidence. Anxiety about an upcoming event is usually based on images of potential disaster; fear of public speaking is a very common example of this type of anxiety. Images of completely losing one's ability to communicate with the audience, or forgetting one's lines, or seeing people shake their heads in disapproval or ridicule, are very powerful. I once had a boss who was a brilliant scientist and dynamic speaker, but could not control his emotions at times. He insisted that I practice my scientific presentations by giving them to him and, during the practice, he would roll his eyes and make sounds of disgust to himself. One time, as I finished a presentation that I was to give three days later, he held his head in his hands and stared at me through his fingers for about twenty seconds before spitting out, "This . . . is . . . a . . . *disaster!*" After going through that a few times, I got so anxious when planning to give scientific presentations that I could feel the tension in my gut for weeks ahead of time.

Many things have changed for me since then, including learning the techniques he taught me, but one of the most significant was that I began to practice imagining the feeling that I was enjoying giving the presentation. First, from the perspective of the audience, I saw myself appearing to be very confident. Then I imagined what it would feel like to be right on top of my game, with the words I wanted coming to me on demand, articulate, connected with the audience, happy to be getting the chance to talk to them, perhaps even sad when the presentation was over. Every time I began to feel anxious about an upcoming presentation, usually as a result of some ghastly image of disaster, I would replace the negative scenario in my mind with the image of feeling confident. The effectiveness of this exercise led me to feel that I was in control of my emotions, which eventually dissipated almost all of my negative emotions about public speaking.

Imagery of emotions in sports is very similar: An anxious athlete can transform her expectations by repeatedly replacing images of disaster with images of the *emotions* that she'll feel when she is fully engaged in her sport. These images will not only reduce performance anxiety, but will also solidify the association between performance and her preferred emotional state while performing. Then, the performance itself will be more likely to elicit the emotions she desires, or at least will remind her to try to access these emotions.

A final application of imagery in sports is its use in motivation toward goals. A friend and colleague of mine in the sports medicine department at Duke was once a world champion weightlifter. Every day for a year he lifted weights for at least three hours. What motivated him to endure this grueling regimen? After all, it's difficult to remain focused on the current task when that task leads to chronic physical pain. Many days, he did not look forward to the experience of training, but what kept him going was the image of being crowned world champion. I'm not in a position to understand this fully, but he has described to me how this image became so emotionally charged for him that he sometimes needed to avoid it for fear of overworking himself and causing injury. It hovered before him each day like a picture attached to a mechanical arm extended in front of his face: Everywhere he looked, it was all he saw. I really don't recommend this; not everyone can be a world champion. But it's impossible to overestimate the power of a very clear, specific reward to motivate someone to work.

Perhaps the most salient result of developing this kind of big image is how an athlete starts to structure his life around the image, to make plans to bring it to life. At times, the image can become so clear that the athlete believes that it's predestined, as though he has glimpsed the future and needs to begin to prepare for it. A successful coach I've worked with wasn't able to reach his goals until he began to live as though he already had. One of the tricky parts of this approach is that it enhances motivation during practice and preparation, but you have to reduce the importance of the big goal while you actually engaged in the activity. LPGA hall-of-famer Beth Daniels once told me that any time she started to rehearse her victory speech while still on the course, she would immediately urge herself to get back to focusing on the golf in front of her.

In a more immediate way, images can generate the motivation for golfers to take the right steps to complete the shot they've seen. While working with golfers on the course, I have asked them to use visualization to prepare to hole a fifty-yard pitch shot. Those who take this task seriously will walk to the green to read the break near the hole; to imagine making the shot, they need to ask themselves the question, how will it get there? In a book called *The Message of a Master*, written by John McDonald in 1929, the author referred to this process as *out-picturing*. The intensity of the internal picture builds like the pressure of a steam engine, and can only be released when it is brought to life, when it is out-pictured, in the external world.

Brain Function and Imagery

ROLAND PERLMUTTER taught me that all brain function is dependent upon velocity. The fundamental feature of brain mechanics is electrochemical messages traveling along neuronal circuits.

"It's all about speed," he told me one day. "The faster the messages can move, the more efficient the brain mechanism will be. Efficiency is crucial in a living organism, since brain size is limited. It may be possible to build a computer the size of a room, but Nature recognized that the brain needs to be portable. So, the most important feature in neuroscience is speed of processing. Any activity that can increase the efficiency of the brain will reduce the time that a process requires, and reduce the amount of brain tissue that has to be carried around in our heads. Increased efficiency in the brain also allows for additional, or more in-depth, processes; you can do more stuff if you need less time to do it. Being totally prepared to do something makes an action easier, more efficient."

"Like priming," I said, referring to the psychological literature on preparing an action.

"That's right. Just as a pump works more efficiently when it's primed, when it's prepared by filling it with whatever liquid it pumps, mental priming can improve the efficiency of brain function."

A lot of studies have demonstrated the effects of priming. For example, research subjects take far less time to find a hidden word when its opposite (e.g., hot *v.* cold) is presented a second earlier. Roland explained that when the neural network involved in finding words of a certain type (in my example, temperature) is stimulated, other words of that type will be found more easily.

"The initiation of action is similarly affected by priming. Imagery primes the brain, reducing the amount of time and effort required to weed out inappropriate or incorrect motor programs and choose the correct ones."

As usual, as Roland talked, he became increasingly animated and excited.

"A number of studies have been done to show how imagery mimics actual movement, and why it may be effective. People have wondered about how the brain imagines for centuries, yet it's only in the past few years that we've had the technology to get a good handle on the differences between imagining movements and actually performing them. Studies suggest that there are several areas of the brain that are active both when we do and when we imagine doing, which may help to explain the effectiveness of imagery: By practicing mentally, we are activating many of the brain regions involved in that action. If imagery is used immediately prior to an action, as in those preshot routines you have golfers do, it primes the proper neural circuits for activity."

Roland pulled out a plastic model of the brain, and went through the different regions that were active during motor imagery and during action. (The figure on page 92 is similar. It includes two pictures of the brain—one from the outside, and an MRI picture showing the side of the brain from the inside.)

"Movement and mental practice are handled by the brain in a very similar way: The supplementary motor area, posterior inferior primary motor cortex, cerebellum, frontal cortex, basal ganglia, and anterior primary motor cortex are all active. Studies done in the 1980s and '90s using PET," he continued, referring to *positron emission tomography*, "were less sensitive than the functional MRI techniques used today. The older PET studies weren't able to find the activation of the motor cortex while people do imagery, so we thought that there wasn't any. However, recent fMRI studies, including some of the studies done here, have repeatedly revealed that when people think about doing something, the brain region responsible for actually doing that action is very active. In fact, some studies have even demonstrated that the cerebellum is mildly active when people imagine themselves doing something. We had always thought that the cerebellum is involved only when actual movement is initiated."

These findings help to explain the power and effectiveness of imagery techniques; they support the idea that seeing is closer to doing than we'd ever expected. Many of the athletes I've worked with who are skeptical about imagery have been impressed by some of the pictures of the brain Roland and his colleagues have provided. They are easily worth the thousand words I would otherwise need to use.

"Obviously, seeing and doing are not exactly the same in the brain," Roland continued, "because one neural process results in the production of actual force, and one does not. Some work has suggested that for imagined actions, the area of activation is broader and less specific than when someone actually moves. Part of this

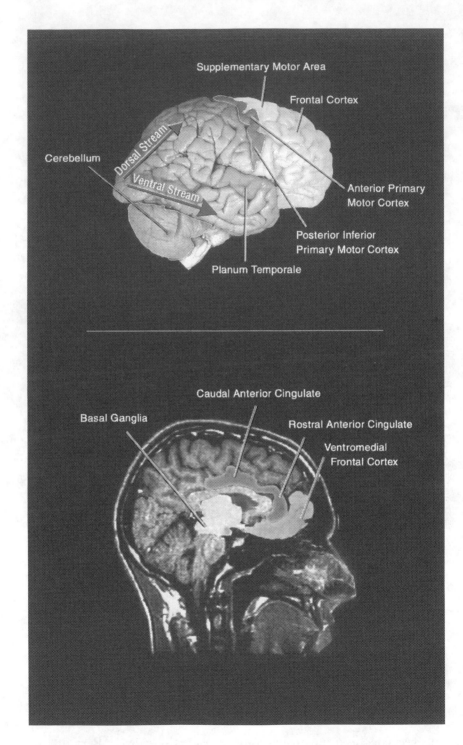

may be due to the fact that people generally do not develop their images with as much detail as they do their plans to actually execute a motor act."

I was familiar with this concept; athletes who had difficulty visualizing always benefited from becoming very specific about the images they were trying to produce, such as reading the writing on the basketball as they imagined themselves holding it in their hands before a free throw. Roland was on a roll, though, so I did not interrupt him.

"Close your eyes," he said.

I closed them.

"Now, say to yourself, 'I imagine moving my hand toward my forehead,' then imagine doing so." I had a vague image of my hand moving, but it was not very clear.

"Now, do it again, except say to yourself 'I am going to move my hand toward my forehead,' and then plan to do so, except stop yourself at the last moment."

I followed his instructions.

"What is the difference?" he asked.

"Well, I noticed that the feeling of the movement is much richer when I actually planned to carry out the action the second time."

"That's right!" he blurted out, punching the air with a finger pointed toward me for emphasis. "What's happening is that the actual plan to carry out an action activates a more specific set of neurons, which results in a more vivid image of the feeling of the movement. There has been a lot of work on why being specific in your intentions leads to more accurate performance. There are two different patterns of visual activity in the brain: the *ventral stream*, which is generally responsible for identifying things in the outside world, like what something is, and the *dorsal stream*, which determines how we interact with those things, such as where something is and what we plan to do about it. These two networks often interact with each other. However, when there is no explicit goal to an imagery task, like the first one you did, the two networks are probably acting independently, each off in its own little world. Imagery that includes a clear intention, a clear goal, is more effective in enhancing performance because it triggers an integration of these two networks. The specific items in the visual field—like the green, the flight of the ball, the feeling of the club—all connect neurally with the plan of action. Sometimes people get very dorsal in their imagery and very ventral when they perform. Imagery that includes more ventral images, which have more specificity, help to integrate the two.

"What's really exciting to me about this work is that it may tell us about the role of consciousness in performance."

I began to have that feeling of standing up in a rowboat listening to Roland. I wanted to hang on to something, not move too quickly, for fear of tipping over. He sped ahead.

"The dorsal system can operate without the awareness of the individual. While the ventral system is very important in identifying things, it can kind of bog down the fluidity of an athlete's play. Being aware of little details like the exact shape of the ball and club are important aspects of the imagery prior to a golf shot, yet they are fairly irrelevant when you're in the middle of hitting the shot. So, an athlete may be unconscious of the details of things in the outside world, yet he will react to these things anyway, without a conscious awareness of what he is responding to. In fact, I'll bet that most of the elite athletes you work with may indeed be able to process a lot of visual information through the dorsal stream. People like Tiger Woods or Michael Jordan, when they're in the zone, are probably very dorsal for brief periods, and their performance surprises even themselves. They perform at the optimal level by not needing to identify what something is before they interact with it. Although you wouldn't want to walk through life this way, such a brain mechanism is very efficient for an athlete."

I had read a paper that described the same thing that Roland was discussing. The authors supported the idea by pointing to the fact that, when athletes talk about their performances, they are rarely able to give a comprehensive verbal account of their best performances, yet can do so when they perform poorly. Knowing all the details of a performance may mean that the athlete was giving too much conscious attention to them. It could also mean that when they perform badly, they try to get better by paying attention to the details.

As Roland described the way in which imagery changes brain function, I became interested in what the long-term effect of imagery may be on the brain. I had instructed a lot of golfers to go through their entire rounds using imagery before each tournament, and had suggested to injured athletes that they visualize themselves moving their injured limb more efficiently and with less pain than they could at the time. I wondered what the long-term effect of this type of mental rehearsal would be on the neural circuits that regulated these functions.

We obviously know that practicing a movement improves the performance of that movement. In one of our initial meetings, Roland told me that practicing an actual movement repeatedly for weeks improves the speed and efficiency of that movement by changing the way the brain is activated when performing it: There is more motor cortex activation and less frontal cortex activation. I asked Roland about how long-term imagery might affect brain function.

"It's a good question," he said. "No one knows. Maybe you should study it and find out."

~

FOLLOWING THESE INITIAL DISCUSSIONS with Roland, my colleagues and I at Duke developed a series of studies that are still being analyzed as this book is written. So far, the findings suggest that imagining a sequence of finger-tapping movements—like pinky, ring, index, middle—for six weeks improved performance significantly compared to not imagining, and was about two-thirds as effective as actually practicing the movements for the same length of time. When we did brain imaging studies on these subjects before and after they had imagined the finger movements for six weeks, the results suggested that, like practice, imagery enhances the ability of a person to carry out an activity quickly and efficiently by increasing the motor cortex's involvement in the task, and reducing the activity of those areas involved in choosing which motor program to complete. As with physical practice, we can improve performance by repeatedly imagining carrying out a task. Yet, unlike physical practice, mental practice can be perfect each time. And since recent studies suggest that neuronal activity generates neuronal connections, this type of practice might actually stimulate brain growth in the regions that are responsible for the activity being imagined.

Present Focus/Concentration

OF COURSE, IMAGERY will only take us so far. Sitting in a room with perfect thinking will not produce much unless we eventually enact our plans. This process is perhaps the most important transition in sports. While broadcasters and commentators may describe the highly tuned athlete as having visions of the championship trophy dancing in his head, at the height of competition most elite athletes are focusing primarily, if not solely, on the task in front of them. Any fears of failure or success are eradicated when the athlete's attention is only on the present. Many professional golfers say the most difficult challenge in winning their first tournament is the distraction of imagining themselves finished with the final round. This future-oriented imagery can disrupt the athlete's concentration on the present. Some of them learn this lesson the hard way: Nick Price has described that when he was twice in a position to win the British Open, each time he began to focus on winning and became certain that he was about to win. In 1982, he had a three-shot lead with a few holes remaining, and became so overly confident and excited that he started severely hooking his drives, and wound up losing to Tom Watson by one shot. It was only after he met several times with sport psychologist Bob Rotella that he became convinced that focusing on the present shot was more effective than urging himself on to win. He won the British Open in 1993.

Imagery can enhance this focus on the present. When the athlete imagines the immediate goal, such as the current shot, instead of the championship, that goal becomes clear and hangs in front of the athlete, and the mind becomes fully absorbed in the task at hand. The image allows the energy of the mind to become quiet and efficient. The motor cortex is primed and ready to do its job on its own. Out-picturing is a process that doesn't involve the frontal cortex's monitoring system, so the athlete feels like she is blending with the moment. This sense of concentration is enhanced further if she allows effortlessness to let action develop from its own spring.

Some athletes use a simple signal to remind them to return to the present. There are two key steps in taking advantage of such a signal. The first is developing the capacity to focus on the present moment and to remember how it felt and how you got there. The second is remembering to use the signal in the height of intense competition. Such a reset button is similar to the trigger of a preshot routine discussed below. It is important for the athlete to practice such a shift in focus repeatedly before using it in competition, so that she'll feel familiar with it and confident that it will be effective.

The signal can be used by an individual for herself or as a team reminder of this state of focus. Several Duke and North Carolina

State teams use such a signal to remind themselves after a poor or excellent play to return to the present, such as slapping the floor to raise intensity on defense or a subtle fist-tap on the hip between plays. The Duke women's lacrosse team developed such a reset signal to remind each other in the height of competition of their support for each other and of their intention to enjoy the process of the game.

Relaxation

AFTER I SPEND TIME working with a golfer on the mental game, I often ask him or her to send me a description of our work together. This not only gets the golfer to rethink our work, but also provides him with a record of what we've done. Quite serendipitously, it keeps me from having to do so. An excellent amateur golfer, who is also a writer, sent me a detailed description of our session, including dialogue. I've never been able to create as good a narrative of working with a golfer on relaxation, so, with his permission, here is his description.

> While I had some control over the process of entering into a state in which the shots seemed to flow out of me, usually the feeling visited briefly and then vanished suddenly. Like a teasing, whimsical lover, the tranquil focus on the present would come to me, yet if I tried to hold on to it or if I expressed any concern over how long it would stay, it was already gone. I had usually tried not to think about it. I often became passive yet covetous, and I reminded myself of a woman I had heard of who claimed that she was sexually involved with a ghost lover who visited her in her bed at night. I waited for the calm to overtake me, yet did not know when it would come or for

how long it would stay. Yet, in my meeting with Dr. Keefe, he seemed to be offering some methods of controlling the capricious wanderings of this mental state.

"I know it feels to you like you don't have much control over when you enter the zone," he said. "Most people feel this way. That's why they attribute its visitation to something outside of themselves, like a magnetic force or a golf god or something. But in reality, it comes and goes based upon things that you do, things that you think. Sport psychologists call them *triggers*. You have a complex set of associations in your brain, and most of the cognitive connections are so complicated that you aren't even aware of them. The trick is to take control of the associative process. If you develop the associations yourself in a conscious way, you can start to have control over when you enter the right mental state. It's like setting up the icons on your computer. Each one represents a whole set of programs that will run whenever you click on it."

He led me over to a bench at the edge of the Duke driving range, where no other golfers were practicing. He instructed me to breathe deeply a few times and took me through a set of relaxation exercises. "Now I want you to allow yourself to focus on how you feel. Let your 'inner observer' watch your thoughts and emotions."

He waited about thirty seconds. "Now look out on to the range and think about how badly you want to hit a great shot." I did this. It was easy for me, as I had this intense feeling of wanting to excel, to succeed, all the time. I felt my pulse increase slightly, and my jaw clenched mildly. I could almost taste my desire, as if I could open my mouth and bite into the external world, chewing on the image of the great shots I would produce.

"Okay, let that image go. Now I want you to relax again.

Focus on your breathing and the relaxation of your muscles like we did before." He paused again for about thirty seconds. "Now, I want you to look out on the range and just look. Have no plan. Let your eyes wander aimlessly over the range without intention. Don't try to remember anything, don't try to absorb anything. Just let your eyes go where they want to. Allow yourself not to try."

I felt the initial wisps of calm come over me. Yet whenever I noticed it, it went away. My doctor seemed to notice this: "You are trying not to try, which interrupts the fluidity of time passing from one moment to the next. It's okay, you'll get better with practice. Let the scene before you intensify and carry you away from the idle chattering in your mind."

Although it was sudden when I noticed it, it had actually come to me quite gradually. I developed an acute awareness of all of the details of the range. The greenness of the grass became alarmingly intense, and I could feel and hear the fluttering of the flags 200 yards away as though they were right next to me. Each view that my eyes came upon seemed to explode with a million different perceptions, and the description of each of them would have required a chapter of verse. I was so captivated by the beauty of what I was seeing, that I had forgotten all about my doctor and what he was doing. My reverie was snapped by the sound of his voice.

"You can see the difference, can't you," he said. I was disappointed to be snatched out of this pleasurable little cocoon, but wanted to hear what he had to say.

"Yes, quite," I answered. "It was very intense, but I felt calm anyway, if that makes any sense."

He nodded and smiled. "It gets a little harder when you have to actually hit a shot, when you have to actually go and do something, but this is the foundation of being able to enter the effortless present whenever you want. The paradox is to have desire yet release it so that you can attain your goal. You must become expert at knowing the difference between the two so that you can alternate between them on the course. You have to become pretty good at it on the practice range if you expect to be able to do it when something important is on the line, like holing a putt to win a tournament."

Preshot Routines

As I MENTIONED, imagery is used at any point before, during, and after an athletic competition. However, at no other time does the athlete have as much opportunity to control, or be controlled by, the impact of his mental state as when he is about to initiate an athletic move outside the flow of action and reaction, such as shooting a free throw, serving in tennis, or hitting any golf shot. These self-initiated acts most benefit from a preshot routine involving imagery. The preshot routine is intended to serve the individual athlete's purposes, so each routine will be different. However, most successful routines include the components described here.

Trigger. The pace of thinking in any sport is vigorous. The athlete is responding to the many physical and mental challenges of his game, and often feels like he is struggling just to keep up, like Lucille Ball on an assembly line. The preshot routine is a way to control the pace of play and the pace of one's thinking. The trigger serves as a dividing line between the frenzy of the sport and the internal peace that best facilitates peak performance. The trigger is a signal that the athlete gives to himself that the routine is about to begin. It is a specific, arbitrary movement, such as tapping the club gently on the ground or pulling on his shirt unnecessarily. It should be a special movement that is not made in any other circumstances and *only* signifies that the routine is about to begin, that the athlete is about to enter the bubble of his *concentration zone.*

The purpose of the trigger is defeated if the athlete chooses a movement that he would make anyway, such as throwing aside a towel before a golf shot or getting the ball from the official prior to a free throw. The act needs to be arbitrary so that it can help the athlete remember to employ the routine. Although this arbitrariness may seem unnecessary, there is a natural tendency of many athletes to forget to use their routines in the crucial situations when they need them most. They become so distracted by the magnitude of the moment that they get off track, so any action that reminds them to enact the preshot routine is helpful. It also aids in making the athlete's approach to the action deliberate. It might sometimes seem easier to let yourself fall into the action, as though you're so relaxed that the shot just sort of happens due to inattention to anything else; this kind of laissez-faire approach may protect the athlete from feeling the pressure of the moment, but it usually doesn't work in crucial situations, when emotional intensity can rise without warning if not controlled proactively.

The trigger, then, in terms of brain function, marks the point of transformation from being a neural system dominated by (1) the vigilant negativity of the anterior cingulate that inhibits inappropriate response choices, and (2) the planning of the prefrontal cortex, to the automatic flow of the motor cortex and cerebellum.

Imagery. As discussed, there are many types of imagery, and any of them can be used as part of the preshot routine. The golfer may see himself from a distance hitting the ideal shot. He may see only the flight of the ball. He may get a kinesthetic image of the swing he wants to make, right through the ball to the top of the finish position. Any of these images can help a golfer, but a focus on just one or two of them is best; the effort to generate images can clutter one's mind as well as anything, and the goal of the preshot routine is to think and try *less*, not more.

For the shooter at the foul line, developing an exact kinesthetic image of the perfect free throw not only primes the brain regions that will initiate this action in a few seconds, but serves as a beacon on which to focus, eliminating all other distractions, internal and external. Usually, a basketball player knows the feeling of a free throw that is released just right, and can call up this image immediately prior to the actual shot. The golfer's images may take a bit more time since, unlike a free throw, each shot is not identical—but the purpose is the same and, once the golfer has a clear image of the shot, it is best to proceed immediately toward its release.

Breath. Initially, this seems like too much to think about during a preshot routine. Why not just allow the breath to take care of itself without all this deliberateness? It's a reasonable question, but a deep breath is an integral component of nearly every successful routine. In crucial situations, the heart rate increases and breathing tends to become shorter and more shallow. These physical manifestations of anxiety not only signal to the athlete that he's nervous, which may further increase his anxiety, but they also deprive the neural systems of needed oxygen. Thus, a deep breath as a matter of course in the routine will ensure that the athlete is at peak condition to initiate the shot regardless of the circumstances. The other aspect of the deep breath is that it keeps the athlete busy. An idle mind allows devilish distractions to interfere with the progression toward releasing the shot. As the athlete goes through the sequence of small activities of the engrained routine, each one follows naturally from the other, without leaving spaces he can fill with thoughts of the circumstances of the action, or the potential disasters that will result from failure. The deep breath is best used at a point in the routine when there is the potential for one of these demonic spaces. With interruption banished, the athlete is like a locomotive barreling down a track, deliberate, forceful, unstoppable in his momentum toward the final expression of the image that he has created.

Spring to life. The final step in the routine is to allow the athletic act to be released from the body. The space just prior to the generation of the movement should be still. There should be no extra effort, no try, no do it or die—just the space, and the reverberating images, and the willingness of the athlete to let his true natural ability come forth. This is the most important moment in sports, and is the moment for which any preshot routine is the preparation. It is the main subject of this book. It is the moment that I originally experienced on that driving range in New Jersey. The shot *arose* from within me. While I had stumbled upon this experience that day, a properly developed and fully engrained preshot routine can make this experience a more regular occurrence.

A full view of the richness of the target aids the feeling of the shot springing to life. In the science-fiction novel *Stranger in a Strange Land* by Robert Heinlein, the wise alien described his culture's focus on completely soaking in all possible information about an object by *grokking* it, which has an implication of not only seeing the perceptible elements of the object, but looking at it so openly and attentively that normally imperceptible elements are understood as well. I think that the last element of the preshot routine before allowing the shot to spring to life should be to *grok* the target. This perception is then so rich that distractions will have no hope of stealing our attention. This is the integration of the dorsal and ventral neural systems that Roland Perlmutter described to me. The next step, that of allowing the shot to spring to life, is then more easily achieved. With no contrasting views, with the image of the shot and the destination in mind, the brain has no choice but to allow the flow of electrochemical circuitry past all of the resistors until the images are released into the external world.

Regular practice of the preshot routine lets you initiate the routine without memory strain or adjustment during an actual game or tournament, but too much practice may render it stale and emotionless. In the preshot routine, the athlete makes the transition from sophisticated human thinker to animal. All of the complex analytic thought that was involved in planning the shot is tremendously important, and the athlete's plans use the full frontal cortex, yet once the trigger is set, a process begins that peels away or diminishes the higher, executive parts of the brain, as the functioning of the brain becomes, by choice, primitive. The athlete is like a lower animal, joined fully with inner and outer nature. There is no more brain activation that we would call thinking, only doing. There is no hesitation. Procession. Reaction. Response. Being.

~

THERE ARE MANY OPPORTUNITIES for athletes to use preshot routines in other sports. The preplay routine in football, particularly for offensive players, is so commonplace that many football players don't even realize that they're engaging in one. The team comes together, receives the play, then usually claps or says a one-word inspirational message, which serves as the trigger. As the players come to the line of scrimmage, their action plans are racing through their neural circuitry, often accompanied by visual and kinesthetic images. With a deep breath, they await the signal that will allow their role in the play to spring to life. Some of my work with football players has been to make this process conscious, so that they can emphasize the components of the routine they need the most. For example, a receiver whose confidence in his hands is waning can rehearse, as he jogs to the line, the image of the ball being gently accepted into his strong and supple hands. The imagery work with a Duke quarterback that I described earlier also included his recalling the imagery through the use of a preplay routine. Such a routine is not limited to offensive players; a defensive end who tends to make impulsive moves to the outside in his pass rush can visualize himself responding to the pass protection by forcing himself inside, or faking the outside rush and then overpowering the offensive line-man in his face. A repeated image of a powerful, immediate response to the snap of the ball, and only to the ball, will facilitate a defensive lineman's quickness and reduce miscues. Even linebackers and defensive backs can use imagery in a preplay routine, seeing them-selves respond correctly to how a play develops in front of them.

The use of a preplay routine for kickers, punters, and long snap-pers is almost essential. The pressures placed on these players is immense, their activity has to be precisely accurate, and mental fac-tors can have a dramatic impact on performance. Furthermore, they usually only receive attention when they make mistakes. Thus, neg-ative images are common, and have to be beaten back with a routine that allows images of success to flourish. A kicker's preplay routine is similar to a golfer's: trigger, image of ball flight, kinesthetic image of the kick, breath, *grok* the target, await the snap that will allow the kick to spring to life. Rhythm is an important element of a kicker's routine too, since he will have to maintain his sequence of motor acts despite the tumult erupting in front of him. He may even need to respond to a poor snap or a penetrating rusher, but he cannot plan that response, or his kick will be thrown off track. He needs to stay completely within his rhythm, stick completely to his plan— aborting it if necessary, but having no thoughts of aborting if *not* necessary.

Self-talk

EVERYONE TALKS TO THEMSELVES. A lot of the sentences are incom-plete, fragmented, and some of them don't make sense. Many of them are critical. We are taught from infancy how to talk to other people, but most people never receive any instruction on how to talk to themselves. I say things to myself that I wouldn't say to my worst enemies. This tendency rarely appears in my everyday life, but for some reason it regularly manifests itself on the golf course. It never helps.

I have always been irritated by the phrase, "If you don't have something nice to say, then don't say anything at all." Sometimes not-nice things need to be said. It may be more effective to say something with a little more vim than, "It upsets me when you let my child play with your loaded gun. . . ." Some people require a concerted effort to be critical when speaking to others—yet when speaking to themselves, they cast aside any hint of kindness. A golfer I know told me, "My 'inner voice' and I have never been properly introduced; he thinks my name is 'asshole.' " What is the effect of this demeaning internal chatter? Well, it's fairly obvious that it doesn't improve performance. We'd get rid of a caddy or partner who spoke to us in this manner. Perhaps we feel that we can't control our own self-talk, so we allow it to continue. However, if we never do anything to interrupt the stream of insults, it's as if we're stuck with an abusive spouse whom we are afraid to leave.

The key to self-talk is reframing the yearning and interest of this inner voice so that revulsion is transformed into promise. The distance between what the self is and what it wants to be is sometimes vast. This manifests itself in words about the lowly nature of the performing self compared to the judging self. The judging self, which talks, creates distance between itself and the scumbag self who has just hit a bad shot. This internal separation of judge and criminal fragments the mind, and impairs performance. Like a child whose parent disavows him if he misbehaves, the performing self becomes isolated, unsupported, and unmotivated. However, if we can use language to join the two selves, the performing self becomes supported and inspired. Talking in terms of *we* often greatly facilitates this union, as in "we can recover here." This way, the judging self acknowledges that the performing self is joined and not separate.

One golfer I know eliminated this separation by interrupting his critical self-talk and saying, "Back to doing," which quieted the critical voice and returned him to a present focus.

Self-talk can also be used to express support. In individual sports like golf and tennis, athletes can use self-talk to encourage themselves or talk themselves out of negativity. The idea of treating oneself like a best friend while performing may seem trite, but it's very effective. Finally, self-talk can remind us to run specific motor programs that don't come naturally. A player on the North Carolina State basketball team who was one of the country's best shooters used to yell out to other players on the foul line, "Flip your wrist," which was the thought that helped him to finish his follow through when shooting free throws. Nick Price used to say to himself "low and slow," just prior to each full shot, which helped him create the image of the right swing path and tempo.

An ideal mental state is one in which there is no separation between selves. However, if the doing and judging aspects of the self are separate, techniques such as self-talk can get them to treat each other better. They reduce the loneliness of the athlete hearing the critical voices that he has ingested over the years. While sport psychologists can help to replace those voices with their support, techniques, and connection, it is ultimately the athlete's relationship with himself that determines whether his athletic activity is painful and ineffective, or successful and filled with joy.

CHAPTER SIX

Golf in the (United) States

Although I was originally loath to see it, my wife had alerted me to the idea that the effortlessness of the experience I had had on the driving range could have meaning beyond golf, beyond sport. The experience itself might even be transformative. The memory of that initial automatic movement was too strong for me to intellectualize away; it still lingers with me years later. Nobel laureate John Nash has said that he believed his bizarre delusions, which focused on aliens taking over the earth, because they came to him in the same revelatory manner as many of his scientific insights. He had come upon brilliant mathematical ideas based upon sudden insight, reaching conclusions never expressed by other people, so it was very difficult for him to dismiss the idea that perhaps he also had insight into a danger to humanity that no one else could see. While I was not legitimately concerned that I had become psychotic, I was aware that a few of the interpretations I was considering could be viewed by others as pretty illogical.

One of these illogical explanations is the possibility that an outside force is actually involved in moving the golf club. Is this reasonable? Well, sort of. In science, all hypotheses are considered; the data are the final arbiters of whether ideas should be accepted or rejected. Absurd hypotheses, of course, are considered and rejected so quickly that it seems as though they are never examined at all.

While I was partially buffeted against rejecting this notion as absurd because so many other seemingly sane people had described similar experiences, it was the sheer power of my memory of the moment that drove me to investigate an idea my academic colleagues would find humorous. I returned to one of my sources of comfort through my many trying intellectual times: Roland Perlmutter.

Although I had known Roland for a while, and he and I had had several conversations about the role of the brain in my experiences, I had never really had the courage to ask him about the possibility that somehow an actual outside force was moving the club, and that I was an observer to the process. This idea, which seemed half crazy only because the other half was stupid, would not go away no matter how much I tried to ignore it or talk myself out of it. Several times when meeting with Roland, I started to bring up the subject of whether the brain could be a vehicle for the interaction between a spiritual force and human experience, but I always backed down, always afraid of extending my intuition too far beyond the safety of my father's automobile and into the world of science. When I considered raising the subject with Roland, I could imagine his eye roll and smirk, then hear him saying, *I'm a world renowned medical scientist giving you my most precious gems, and you bring up spirituality and half-baked mysticism? Go back to your little sport psychology world! I'm talking about* real *science here! Get the hell out of our medical center, and take your petty little brain with you!*

One evening, when I was working late on some of the data from a brain imaging project, I ran into Roland in the parking lot. Spring had come early that year, and the warm evening air reminded me that soon the evenings would be longer and after-work golf would again become a possibility. I was feeling discouraged by a full day of brain-imaging data analyses that hadn't yielded any of the findings I expected and, despite the weather, I felt gloomy. Roland was taking the pleasant spring air more to heart, and was gazing at the night sky when I approached him.

"The heavens," he said, waving an unfolding arm through the air.

"I'd settle for one," I replied, somewhat surprised by my own expression of discouragement. I didn't know if I was faking humility or was just tired from being in front of a computer all day.

"Still working on that data set?" he asked, sensitive to my frustration with the analyses.

"Well, we made a mistake in the design of the study, so the computer has to work hard to try to make up for it. I keep hoping to find that our mistake was actually higher intuition in disguise, but it doesn't seem to be so far."

"You try too hard sometimes," he said bluntly. "It's not all in your hands, you know."

I was surprised he would ascribe agency outside me, and wondered if he was referring to chance or something else. I thought of seizing the opportunity to discuss the possibility of an actual spiritual force, then suddenly and defensively switched directions. "I suppose I should just 'give it up to God,' " I said, knowing I was mocking something I had considered. I had a sudden image of a friend of mine who as a child had been so embarrassed by his mother's thick Spanish accent at a parent–student meeting that, when a friend asked him who she was, he denied knowing her. I felt the same, like I was denying something close to my heart, and that I had placed myself in the position of arguing on the exact opposite side of where I wanted to be.

"It's probably not that simple, Rich," he replied, seeming a little stung.

"I know, I know," I said, shaking my head and looking down, "I've just been so frustrated with this project; it seems to be going on forever," sticking with discouragement as an excuse for my apparent pessimism, which had more to do with the vulnerability I felt when I began to consider spiritual explanations for anything. "It really doesn't feel like inspired exploration these days, more like work."

Roland operated interpersonally on a different level from most people. He sometimes seemed to change the subject dramatically, and only in retrospect could you see that he had been answering the question that you did not yet realize you had. He paused and looked pensive.

"It's funny; I gave a lecture the other day on my research on automatic, effortless movements to a group of basic scientists down the road at Chapel Hill. It was on the main campus, away from the medical center, and a couple of people from the religion department showed up. An older fellow stood up and described how Buddhist and Christian monks focus their whole lives on having experiences that seem to be driven by a higher power. He said that the Christians feel it is God working through them and the Buddhists feel it is the highest form of enlightenment. He said there was something basic and fundamental through all cultures about these types of automatic experiences, and that most cultures found them to be tremendously important. It was fascinating. A couple of people in the audience started asking *him* questions, and it led to a pretty intense argument, in which one group was insisting that these experiences were directed by God, while the other group believed that the experiences were nothing more than a quirk in the organization of the brain. Finally, the old guy said, 'I think we're all describing the same elephant here,' you know, referring to the old analogy of blind men rubbing different parts of an elephant and trying to understand what it is. 'If there is a God, and spiritual experience is available to us, there needs to be some kind of mechanism through which we gain access to it. The brain would certainly be a likely candidate! And Dr. Perlmutter's research seems to be giving us an idea of how the brain opens a window for us to allow the glory of God's light to shine upon us.' "

I gulped hard, wanting to scream, *That's what I've been trying to ask you for a couple of years!* I felt a bizarre mixture of tremendous excitement about not being completely alone in considering the connection between brain function, athletic performance, and spiritual experience, and a horrible fear that my insecurity about asking such questions would keep me from a full understanding of the experiences I had had. My fear had the effect of coloring my excitement toward panic, and I felt I needed to do something immediately in order to experience that transcendence again. I also felt a resolve forming in my mind and, as it grew, my panic lessened: I knew I needed to find the larger relevance of the experience I had had, no matter how crazy or stupid it seemed.

I looked up to ask Roland what he thought of that, but he was already in his car, waving as he pulled away.

Our Limited Interpretations of Experience and Possibility

IN WESTERN CULTURES, the idea that an external force acts upon us is usually discussed by referring to God. The term *God* means different things to different people, and I hesitate to define it here since I am certainly not an expert in theology; I have many more questions, hopes, and dreams than I do answers in this arena. When I use the term *God* I mean a universal, spiritual force that exists outside of humans as well as interacting with them. The benevolence of this force is implied, but not certain.

Does God govern our games? The most common argument against this idea is that, even if there is such an outside force, it must be too busy or have better things to do than to be concerned with the outcome of our petty little sports events. Every year, around the time of the Super Bowl, magazine articles note that a surprisingly large percentage of players in the game will pray for God to have an impact on the game in various ways, from asking for God's will to be expressed through them, to asking for God to choose their side to win. This view is condescendingly criticized by esteemed theologians and slyly mocked by the writers of the articles. Yet in this position lies the arrogance of ignorance; we have enough trouble understanding the mechanisms of our own experience, so how can we understand the limitations of the divine? If there is some kind of universal force that affects our lives, and if it is all-knowing and all else that this implies, the attention span of this power might well be a little more developed than mine, and it could well have the capacity to work on the problems of hungry children on the planet, the pining of lovers at the beach, and the kink in my backswing, all at the same time.

Most of us place tremendous limitations on possibility. The earth seemed flat, so it was deemed to be so. The sun seemed to revolve around our planet, so it became sacrilege to think otherwise. Even our creative fiction reflects this limitation: Almost all of the life forms in science-fiction novels, even those created by the best writers, are humanoid, with human perspectives. Surely there are other evolutionary paths in the universe. Every organism perceives only a tiny fraction of the available data from the universe. Why would humans be different? Why would our development as a species have included every possible aspect of perception? There are many examples on earth of species that can perceive aspects of reality that humans cannot. Consider the auditory and visual systems of bats; most are unable to perceive light, yet with the use of a highly developed system of echolocation, they can maneuver through a dark nighttime world that two short centuries ago was completely unavailable to us. It is almost impossible to imagine what it would be like to actually *be* a bat, since their internal world is so different from ours. Are there other aspects of reality that we don't perceive, or, like a bat that sees with a form of sonar, that we do not perceive directly? It is difficult to get far enough outside our notion of experience to imagine such an experience. We always come back to ourselves as the standard: If we do not experience it, we figure, it must not be true. How could the earth be anything but flat?

Polls conducted in the United States suggest that about 95 percent of the population believes in God as a force greater than us that guides our lives. How people see this God differs substantially, from a big man sitting somewhere up in the sky to a process in the universe that governs life or interacts with it without playing favorites, as gravity imposes its will on objects based only on their mass. I know some very smart people who believe in God, but it seems that most people who are known for their intelligence deny the existence of a spiritual force in the world. Sometimes this troubles me. If I interpret certain events and feelings in my life as suggesting a process or a power beyond me, is it just a reflection of my limited cognitive abilities?

I had a discussion about divine intervention with one of my brightest colleagues, who is also a good friend. He is well known to people in brain research for his ability to solve complex problems, and he loves to discuss his ideas on any subject. One night at a bar, during a scientific conference, I told him that I was troubled by the experience I had had of the golf club moving on its own, and asked him to consider that possibility that some kind of spiritual force somehow interacts with the events of our daily lives. He pulled no punches.

"I realized when I was five years old that God did not exist," he said, unaware or unconcerned that he was comparing my current intellectual capacity with his before age five. "It seems pretty obvious to me that the whole notion of God developed as a way to help people face the misery of their lives. The chances of any of that being true are astronomically small."

I tried different arguments to penetrate the walls of the fortress he had erected around his disbelief, but I was swiftly refuted each time. When our fourth round of drinks was delivered, I realized that

God is an excellent topic for the second and third rounds at a bar, but that efforts to understand more about the divine become futile thereafter. I switched the topic to sex.

The next morning, after having missed a few of the early presentations, I shook off my hangover and headed into a talk on the effects of different medications on brain function. I saw my friend again, and sat next to him. He had been to all of the early talks, which impressed me. "You gotta play hurt," he said with a chuckle.

As my mind wandered during the presentation, I found myself repeating the words *play hurt* over and over. I looked over at him as he soaked in all of the data that were being presented; occasionally he whispered an insightful comment about the weaknesses in the design of a study or referred to the contrast between these results and others that he had seen. He was brilliant, for certain, but he was also unhappy, injured. He played hurt. How does a five-year-old decide that spiritual life is folly? I realized that I did not know him well enough to challenge him fully on his beliefs about God. Religious beliefs are indeed personal, based upon who we were and how that led up to who we are. I did not agree with my friend, and I did not really understand him. And while I respected his intellect and his opinions, I sensed that something had gone wrong many years ago. His complete denial of the possibility of a divine power in the world was not necessarily due to his superior intelligence, but perhaps both of them were due to something else. Perhaps he had been taught early lessons about faith's disappointments, and had constructed an edifice of logic against ever feeling that loss again. I don't know, but it made me wonder about the choices that we make regarding happiness and truth. *Is it better to be wrong and happy, or right and unhappy?*

Depression is associated with seeing oneself more clearly. Research with people who are depressed suggests that they are more likely to evaluate their performance on mental tasks, such as remembering phone numbers, more accurately than people who are not depressed. Is this because a person who sees the truth about herself is unable to overlook her deficiencies, and is therefore more likely to become inconsolably bleak about the dearth of future prospects? Or does the depressed state itself alter her ability to judge herself with the inaccuracy of optimism? Perhaps there is a third alternative. Perhaps failed hope and optimism, especially early in life, discourage faith. Better to know the truth, and to invest only in what is evident, than to raise hope and risk disappointment. A lifetime of this strategy may be rewarded with a greater accumulation of facts and even a superior penchant for understanding mechanisms, but the cost is tremendous: Past failure is taken as an indication of things to come. There are no brand new days, no bright horizons looming gracefully off in the distance. There is no feeling of the possibilities bursting out of each moment. A depressed coach once said to me after the first half of the season was completed, "This season is a disaster; there is no happy ending for us. That only happens in fantasies and Hollywood movies. We are finished." With half of the season still to play, the coach literally could not see a future; she could only see the past.

While this type of belief system is extreme in people with depression, many people who are not clinically depressed have it in a milder form. Psychologist Martin Seligman referred to this common state as *learned helplessness,* meaning that some people develop a sense of being pushed and shoved by the cruel exigencies of life to the point that they feel as though they cannot affect the outcome. They have learned to be helpless. "Anything I do is met with failure," their thinking runs, "so why try?" The result of this type of thinking is an extreme constriction of the experience of possibility. Laboratory and real-world research has indicated that people who begin to experience helplessness dwell on the experience of past failures to the point that they have no mental resources available for planning for the future. Any plans they do make are stunted, immature, and ineffective. This process further inhibits any spark that might open them up to possible alternative interpretations of the world around them. The future holds failure because the past was wrought with it: "If a spiritual force were guiding me, why did it lead me down such sullen pathways? When I swing a golf club, I am alone in my efforts, which usually fail. Any comfort that I feel by a presence with me while I walk or play is merely an illusion designed to generate hope that will later be destroyed." Faith is risky.

Solidly on the other side of the spectrum of "openness to alternative interpretations of golf experiences" are Michael Murphy and his mythological golf pro/guru, Shivas Irons. Murphy's influential story about his spiritual experiences on a golf course in the United Kingdom, written in 1972, was very popular, which surprised even Murphy. Twenty years after *Golf in the Kingdom* was published, Murphy wrote a huge tome on the mind-body connection, entitled *The Future of the Body*. During his speaking tour to promote his book, he found that question-and-answer sessions were entirely devoted to questions about Shivas Irons. Something about this premise moves us: Golfers, more than any other athletes, are able to see their sport as a podium for spirit.

Golf in the Kingdom has developed a cult following substantial enough to challenge *The Rocky Horror Picture Show*. There are about 1,500 members of the Shivas Irons Society, which is named to honor the protagonist in Michael Murphy's classic novel. Like the reenactments of *Rocky Horror*, members get together to play golf, sing, wax poetic, and drink whiskey like the characters in the novel. Some even dress as Scottish golfers from the 1800s and play with a baffing spoon and featherie. Sheepishly, I must admit that I am a dues-paying member of this group. I also once wrote an article for their newsletter, and have played golf with the founder, Steve Cohen, who is a fine man. Although I was once invited to speak at one of their events, I have never attended one. I would expect that there is a strong hope among the attendees that the spirit of Shivas Irons will appear, and transform average golfers into enlightened masters, if only for one hole, one shot.

One of the most illuminating aspects of the Shivas Irons phenomenon is that the author says he doesn't understand the second half of the book. Perhaps the truth of these experiences is less important to some people than the fact that other people share them. It is nice not to feel alone, especially when we have strange interpretations of the world around us. Although the book does little to provide explanations for spiritual experiences in golf, there is something appealing about the idea of a guru taking us and teaching us about spirituality—and we get to play golf at the same time! In some parts of the book, the character Shivas Irons speaks with such a heavy Scottish accent that it is difficult to understand what he is saying; this too may be part of the appeal to people—the presence of someone foreign and slightly incoherent probing the nature of our souls. In some ways, the character reminds me of a woman reading a crystal ball: Once the stage is set and you go into the dimly lit room with curtains everywhere, a glowing orb, and a strange woman with jet-black hair staring at you intensely, anything she says will seem to have a lot of merit. I've always wondered whether the popularity of other modern gurus in the United States didn't stem somehow from their looking different than the average American. Would Deepak Chopra have sold as many books and calendars if his name were Bob? (This of course makes the balding Wayne Dyer's popularity even more impressive, though it was jumpstarted when people mistakenly thought they were going to learn about sex and orgasm from the title of his first popular book, *Your Erroneous Zones*.) It is when the person instructing us is *other* that we feel that they know more; to be like us would make them deficient. Even though they discuss a journey toward the *self*, they are only appealing to us if they imply a promise that they will take us away from ourselves. Despite my skepticism about Murphy's book, I enjoyed reading it, and it encouraged me that my experiences were something that I shouldn't try to ignore.

Mystical Experience

THE EXPERIENCE of a golf club moving on its own could be described as *mystical*, although I cringe at the use of this term. My embarrassment is not really about the nature of my experiences, but is due to the fact that the term *mystic* and its derivations (mystical, mysticism) are so seriously misunderstood. People associate the word *mystical* with *mysterious* and believe that an essential element of mysticism is the unknown or bizarre. The prototypical representation of this misunderstanding is the wizard in the tall cone-shaped hat covered with stars, moons, and astrological signs. Yet the consideration of mysticism in golf and other sports is not an astrological endeavor; it's an exploration of how changes in one's mental state can make someone feel that something larger than him is somehow joining with him.

Surveys in the United States, Britain, and Australia find that between 20 and 40 percent of people report having had mystical experiences. In a study by sociologist Robert Wuthnow, about half of 1000 randomly selected individuals reported having experiences involving "contact with the sacred," and 39 percent reported having experienced being in harmony with the universe. Granted, Wuthnow's research took place in Berkeley in the early 1970s, but more recent research has supported the idea that a large minority, if not a majority, of people have had experiences similar to mine. If my experience was indeed weird, at least it was not abnormal.

I was fortunate that this type of experience has been described by eloquent authors for thousands of years. One of the grandfathers of modern psychology, William James, reviewed these writings about a hundred years ago. He described mystical states as ineffable, noetic, transient, and passive. This description may require a bit of further explanation. First, *ineffable* means beyond words. Mystical states are so powerful and overwhelming that language seems to be a weak vehicle for communicating about them to other people. Some people have devoted their lives to trying to do so. Second, the *noetic* nature of mystical states refers to the experience that important new knowledge is being acquired. They are not just feelings that arise; the experience results in conclusions about the nature of reality. Third, the experience is *transient* in that it usually lasts no longer than an hour or two. Finally, although mystical states can be attained through preliminary voluntary operations, such as meditation or prayer, when the consciousness has begun, the person feels *passive*, as if her own will has dissolved, replaced by a power external to it, sometimes as if she were grasped and held by a superior power.

It was the last of these characteristics that most caught my attention. I had read a number of original narratives of experiences that describe this aspect of mysticism, and it seemed that each religion interpreted the experience differently. For Christians, the contact with an external power is usually God, or Christ. The Christian mystic feels God's will in his movements, thoughts, feelings, and impulses; it is described as blissful and transformative. Other religions interpret these experiences in different ways, but all of them hold the mystical experience as the pinnacle of spiritual life. Buddhism and Hinduism describe *Nirvana* as a level of spiritual awakening in which the individual's consciousness becomes completely integrated with the greater consciousness of the universe. This experience is also blissful, yet the external something is not interpreted as God, especially in Buddhism, since God is not a part of the Buddhist belief system. There are also numerous varieties of nonreligious mystical experience, including those precipitated by nature, ingested substances, athletic activity, and even psychosis.

Is there some kind of unifying principle in these experiences across different religions and cultures? Is this experience really a penetration into the realm of the divine? Or is it a psychological alteration? Is the experience a truth, or a delusion? If it is a truth, what is it? If it's a delusion, why is it universal? It seemed to me that one way to make this determination would be to find the common principles of these experiences across the world, then explore those experiences in terms of psychology and brain science. This became a bit of a bootstrap operation, however. The common elements of mystical experience are elusive, since the experiences themselves are interpreted and described in the context of the individual's belief system. A Christian who, in the midst of prayer, feels her concerns for her own needs disintegrate and is awakened to a feeling of love for others and devotion to their well-being, will interpret this experience as the intervention of God; a Buddhist who enters the same mental state would not include God as a fundamental component. Those who have mystical experiences outside the context of religion have the most difficulty describing their experiences, and are most likely to refer to them as ineffable. The brain does not have a template for experiences unknown to it; if you had never worn a coat, why would you build a coat rack?

I was initially disheartened by the tendency of mystics to interpret their experiences in terms of their past. It seemed so human. If the mystical moment is transcendent, then shouldn't the mystic move beyond the limitations of his history toward something universal? It reminded me of my own limitations when I'm driving from a place I've never been to a place I know well: I always try to get back to a familiar area, then take a route that I've taken many times before. (Some of my trips have consumed far too much time as a result of these hairpin-shaped routes; an overview of where I am and where I am going, along with the courage to delve into the unfamiliar, would have kept a substantial amount of exhaust from being blown into the Research Triangle.)

The human brain traces history selectively. Our memories are the building blocks for interpreting future experiences, but those memories are adulterated, not pure. For the most part, our memory serves us well; we learn that automobiles can crush our bodies, so we stay out of the street and, except for a brief period of denial from ages sixteen to seventeen, we hold to that belief. Our memory in this regard keeps us alive. However, there are instances in which the selectivity of our learning handicaps us. Recent brain-imaging studies suggest that trauma during childhood, especially sexual trauma, actually changes the structure of the brain. We used to think that people were born with all the neurons their brains would ever have, but in 1999, what Roland had referred to as *scientific gossip* was published, demonstrating that the adult primate brain can actually generate new brain cells. Different types of experience lead to different types of neurogenesis: Increased learning will result in new growth of neurons in the brain regions responsible for learning and memory, while in people with a history of trauma, the traumatic experience is so important that the brain develops in a unique way to adapt to it. Why this happens is still unclear, but presumably the brain has mechanisms for accommodating all kinds of different experiences. Parts of the brain involved in memory, such as the superior temporal gyrus, are larger in people who experienced trauma. Their frontal cortex, which serves many functions, including a kind of executive role in the brain, is smaller. The corpus callosum, which transfers information back and forth between the left and right hemispheres, is also smaller. One interpretation of this pattern of brain differences is that people who have experienced trauma develop a brain system that remembers the traumatic event very, very well, but it is cordoned off from the rest of the brain so that it will not be accessed. Even the analytic, decision-making aspects of the brain are diminished, perhaps as a by-product of this banishing of memory, or perhaps as a result of the traumatized person's desire to reduce access to what has been tucked away in the recesses of recognition. One caveat to this research is that these studies have only compared people with trauma to people without trauma; it could be that the brains of the people who were traumatized were different even before the trauma. However, some studies have shown that children who have been abused do not have the same rate of brain development as those who haven't, so it seems fairly likely that the traumatic event is having an impact on their brain.

(An interesting sidelight on how the brain grows in adults is that recent research suggests that drugs like fluoxetine [known as Prozac], which serve ultimately to disinhibit the transmission of the neurochemical serotonin in the brain, may decrease depression by increasing neurogenesis. Thus, depression may be caused by [or causes] brain-cell death; these medications may somehow reverse this process.)

Experiments conducted with animals underscore the conclusion that both adult human brain growth and the interpretation of current experience are determined by past experience. A cat raised in a laboratory that includes only stark black-and-white vertical lines will be completely unable to perceive the horizontal aspects of objects. Even though its eyes operate normally, the visual centers of its brain lack the neural pathways for perceiving horizontalness; it will repeatedly bump into horizontal surfaces, such as tabletops, unless it turns its head ninety degrees to the side. The human brain may be even more sensitive to past experience. Our complex understanding of the natural and social world in which we live is constantly being updated by the lessons we learn as we navigate through time. Each of these lessons alters our brain and, thus, alters how we interpret the next lesson. To continue with the example of the impact of traumatic experience, some people who have been traumatized tend to see trauma everywhere. In extreme cases, the person who has been sexually abused as a child later sees other adult-child interactions as somehow abusive, even to the point of reporting innocent adults to child protection services. Rather than know what we see, we tend to see what we know.

Despite the human neural limitation of being unable to understand the present without the context of the past, and the vast differences among the cultures and religions in which mystical experiences arise, there is a common theme of unity among the various interpretations of the experience. In normal everyday life, we feel our isolation and separateness from the outside world. We usually feel a boundary between the world inside our skin, where we think and feel, and the outside world of people and things. In the throes of a mystical experience, however, a person feels completely united with the world outside, losing his sense of self. While this could be terrifying outside the context of mystical experience, and can occur in psychotic states, in mystical experiences it is blissful. The mystic feels a complete absorption with the *other*, whether that *other* is God, the universe, nature, or another important element of the person's belief system. The elimination of the boundary between self and other is not only ecstatic, but it almost always leads to a transformation of the person's life. Since mystical states often include experiencing contact with a force that is divine and all-knowing, the person emerges with a reduced concern for personal matters, and a greatly enhanced focus on the needs of others.

"When is a man in mere understanding?" German mystic Meister Eckhardt wrote in the early fourteenth century. "When a man sees one thing separated from another. And when is he above mere understanding? When he sees all in all." To see the club and my hands and the tee and the flight of the ball and its destination against the net is to see division. For the brief minute before I interrupted my reverie by calling my wife, there was no separateness among these things: The club had been swung and the ball had been launched; the *I* who held the club was not divisible from the club and its movement. It felt like an outside force was acting through me.

There was no future or past, only the present. The swing, the path of the ball, and its target were all together as one, outside of anything that we call time.

St. Teresa, St. John of the Cross, and the Greek mystic Plotinus experienced such an outside force as God. "It was granted to me to perceive in one instant how all things are seen and contained in God," St. Teresa wrote. "I did not perceive them in their proper form, and nevertheless the view I had of them was of a sovereign clearness and has remained vividly impressed on my soul." My soul was impressed as well. I had opened a door. Perhaps my request to have the club swing itself had been heard by some kind of universal cosmic consciousness that operated in a manner I could not understand. I had asked for the club to move on its own and my request was granted. Perhaps I had connected with something that people have called God. I felt special and arrogant and foolish all at the same time. It is difficult even to think about, let alone write about. Who was I to doubt that God could have acted through me? Who was I to expect that God *would* have acted through me? Perhaps I had not felt a force acting through me at all; perhaps my memory has accentuated some aspect of the experience that was only faintly present. Perhaps I have become more impressed with the experience over time because my neurons reorganized themselves around this illusion. I began to doubt what had happened to me. As time went on, I felt that I was at a crossing point, a fork in the road: I could abandon my search, or continue on with the faith that the meaning I remembered was true.

Reading the experiences of others was partially reassuring. On the one hand, many mystics had been respected members of their church or temple, even writers or philosophers. On the other hand, I ran across a medical literature associating religious experiences with epilepsy. There are several forms of epilepsy, and some of them greatly increase the likelihood that the afflicted person will have mystical or religious experiences. An impressive number of religious leaders and prophets have been documented to have epilepsy, among them Muhammad, Joan of Arc, Joseph Smith, and even Saint Paul. Some medical circles continue to refer to epilepsy as "Saint Paul's disease."

While I considered that maybe I had some form of incipient epilepsy, I realized that the two don't always go hand in hand. The problem with so-called abnormal experiences, as described by medical professionals, is that people who go to their doctor are by definition suffering. If someone is having seizures, which is certainly a problem, and these seizures are associated with religious experiences, then the experiences themselves will be associated with the seizures, which is the problem that compelled them to go to a doctor. What about people who have the same experiences but aren't suffering? Since they do not seek treatment, they're absent from the medical literature.

The human nervous system is designed to allow a vast array of behaviors and experiences. It is often the context of the experience that determines whether it's problematic or adaptive. Evidently, the brain has available to it the capacity to experience a feeling of oneness with the outside world, to feel the presence of an external force, to be filled with bliss. The fact that these can occur prior to, or during, the frenzied electrical concert of a brain seizure does not mean they are limited to this particular cause. If about half of all people have some experience of direct contact with the divine or feel a oneness with the outside world, and less than 1 percent of people have seizures, there must be more to these experiences than a potential brain disorder. The brain is not a rigid structure with all parts occupying a specific place and function like an automobile engine; it is designed to be structurally and functionally flexible. It has a multitude of potential operations, many of which can either be adaptive or maladaptive depending upon the situation. The haywire brain can have spiritual experiences, but this doesn't mean that St. John, Jesus, Buddha, and the monk on the mountaintop all had haywire brains. It most likely means that the capacity expressed in the experiences of these religious people is also expressed in the person with epilepsy, though in the latter the experience is disorganized, dysfunctional, and out of control.

I wondered how far back in history people have had these experiences. To feel the oneness with the other, whether that other is God or nature or another aspect of universal consciousness, it's essential to have first felt separate from these things. Without consciousness of the self, the dissolution of this boundary is impossible, since there is no boundary. Before we were able to look at ourselves, before we were able to examine what we did or thought, we were incapable of feeling the separation between ourselves and the rest of the world. We only longed for the Garden of Eden when we were kicked out; before that, it was just home. Yet, that sweet scent of home lingers in the way our genes distribute our neurons as we develop in the womb; the longing for reunion is present in all of us. I felt as though, for a minute, that longing in me had been quenched.

I generally don't take the Bible literally, but it occurred to me very strongly that one day long ago, there was an Adam. For the first time, a primate looked at himself (or herself) and criticized what he saw. "How do I work this?" he thought. Soon after, he said, "I can do better." He now had a tremendous advantage over everyone else, as he could improve himself. He would transmit to his progeny this ability to view himself and improve himself and, as the eons passed, they would conquer the earth. Little did Adam know when he first saw in himself something that needed work, that scores of millennia later our hands would shake as we imagined what our fellow golfers might think of us while we stand over the ball on the first tee.

In the brief moment on the practice tee in New Jersey, I had not monitored my performance. I did not say to myself, "I hope this works." I did not try to force myself into the unfolding of the swing. I did not struggle. I did not strain. I allowed the swing to arise. I allowed the ball to be released. As it hovered on the rubber tee, it was like an equals sign in a mathematical formula: On one side of the equation was my swing, on the other was the powerful, gentle arch of the flight of the ball. I felt as though I could no more change the swing or the result than I could change the nature of mathematical principles. This connection between me and the event was so fluid and uninterrupted, that it was as though I were no more there than I was everywhere. The perfection of the swing and the ball flight and the moment were imperturbable. The oneness of the swing and swinger was complete, and this united state produced a perfect result.

This unity between observer and observed is described symbolically as the reunion of God and human before Adam's fall. The act is not made unconsciously, but with consciousness suspended; we allow our powerful mental operations for monitoring ourselves to lie dormant. When we act without the internal pressure of desire, the action and the actor are one. The road bends and the car turns; the movement of our hands on the steering wheel is unnoticeable. In our current world, which values self-consciousness more than in any time in history, the merging of self and divine is ever rarer, and ever sweeter.

~

THE MYSTIC WHO experiences God is usually alone; the presence that accompanies her and permeates her moments generally comes to her when she can focus on it completely. We are also solitary in our golf; no one hits the shot but us, and any interference or aid other than the advice of a caddie is against the rules. The feeling of standing over a shot is lonely. The outcome, the process, the initiation of the swing, are all up to us. In other sports, a player may feel alone—bringing the ball up court in the closing seconds of a tight game against North Carolina at the Dean Dome can be very lonely—but the player has his teammates and coaches and the ten people from the visiting team who are given tickets to join with him in the struggle. When attempting to hit a three-wood into a right-to-left green with water right and OB left, there are no teammates and coaches to console you or embrace you if you fail or if you succeed. It is important to realize, at this point, that only in our aloneness are we still enough to open ourselves up to the presence of something greater than ourselves.

"Alone and identity and the mood," Walt Whitman wrote, "and the soul emerges, and all statements, churches, sermons, melt away like vapors. Alone, and silent thought, and awe, and aspiration—and then the interior consciousness, like a hitherto unseen inscription, in magic ink, beams out its wondrous lives to the sense. Bibles may convey and priests expound, but it is exclusively for the noiseless operation of one's isolated Self to enter the pure ether of veneration, reach the divine levels, and commune with the unutterable."

It is when they are the most alone that people are most compelled to invite a divine presence into their lives. This invitation may come as a request to change a fundamental aspect of their being, or it may come as a desire to have help with the moment. I have heard theologians argue that these invitations are always answered; no request goes ignored, but the response is sometimes hard to decode. When the connection to the presence is made, however, no interpretation is needed.

The mystic feels passive in the throes of the experience, as though she is an agent of divine intervention. One reason that many of us have difficulty with this type of consciousness is that we object to being passive. We are taught to strive, to assert, to conquer. We fear that, in waiting for the soul to "emerge," as Whitman says, we risk losing our individuality and falling prey to the meanderings of the group consciousness or to destructive others. We also lack the patience to wait for the moment to come; we try to initiate it before the opportunity is lost. We need to *do* something. The reason our watched pot never boils is that we get so tired of waiting passively, that we get up and kick over the son of a bitch! The mystic waits for an outside agency to initiate her actions, and feels this power move her along. Time itself seems to be irrelevant as each moment flows gracefully, continuously, into the next and the next and the next.

One of the most fascinating aspects of this literature is that this focus on others is not only found in people who have devoted their lives to their religion, such as Christian and Buddhist monks, but also in those for whom mystical experience was a complete surprise. It was as though the shift of attention from self to other was the *point* of the experience. A man with a heavy heart goes out in the morning for a twenty-minute jog, and comes back feeling as though something had been moving his body forward, compelling him, supporting him. It is like a scientist finding evidence of extraterrestrial life; he will never look at his own life in the same way again.

While I felt compelled to explore the nature of my experience on the driving range, I was sometimes burdened by the superficiality of the surroundings. If I was going to have an experience of the divine, shouldn't the circumstances be slightly more hallowed than hitting range balls off of a rubber tee on landfill in New Jersey? The possibility that I had somehow accessed a universal consciousness was wonderful; the fact that it had occurred in the context of golf was fairly perturbing. I was going to have trouble communicating the profundity of the moment to the nongolfers in my life, which consisted of almost everyone I knew. I had visited dozens of other places that seemed more likely to precipitate such an experience: Jerusalem, the Church of the Holy Sepulchre, the Dome of the Rock, the Grand Canyon, the Vatican, even Malibu. I had visited some of these with the specific intent of making contact with the divine, and any of those settings would have made for a perfectly sensible story to share with friends, family, and colleagues. And, if the experience had to be golf-related, why couldn't it be in St. Andrews or Pebble Beach? No. My contact with what may have been a force greater than I came on a landfill, practicing golf when I should have been at work researching mental illness. How could I dare tell anyone other than my wife?

CHAPTER SEVEN

Death Grip

For YEARS, I HAVE HAD a recurring dream of being pursued by an angry gang of young native men in a foreign country. They are wielding machetes, and trying to cut off my hands. I awake terrified, almost too afraid to move. As consciousness returns, I often wonder what it would be like to live with such a fear of death and mutilation, and worse, to constantly fear the same for my children. Then, suddenly, the relative meaninglessness of my golf rushes in like a winter wind. Especially in these times of global uncertainty, golf—with its lush greenery, expanses of open land, and its country club, out of harm's way associations—seems almost unpatriotic in its extravagance.

At these times, I feel guilty for allowing myself the pleasure and peace of playing golf, and I view my interest in understanding all that I've experienced in the game as worthless, perhaps even disturbed. I think not only of the billions of needy people across the world, but also of the needs of those in my own neighborhood, hospital, and home. The meaning that I've found in golf and my desire to understand more about it vanishes, and I am left wondering how I ventured so far down this path. Reflecting on the altruism that followed from the mystical experiences of others, I feel isolated and embarrassed.

Losing Meaning

EVEN IN THE STILLNESS of the water, before nature's tumult distorts our image, our reflection is difficult to bring into focus. I was raised without real exposure to war, turning eighteen in 1976. My age group was the only one since 1948 not to have to register for a military draft. By the age of twenty-five, my father, uncle, and brother had all experienced war directly: My father flew missions over Italy in World War II; my uncle was killed in training. My brother, born in 1951, suffered the conflict of our nation with his generation's war in Vietnam. I have been sheltered from war and, as a young man, I struggled to find meaning in its absence.

Creating meaning in a time without an immediate call was a challenge. I remember volunteering in a soup kitchen in New York City in the early 1980s; I did it a few times until I felt that some of the people who were coming in for free meals had more money than I did. I began questioning whether what I was doing was really good for others. I never really answered the question, but I figured that, if I wasn't deriving any satisfaction from the effort, and felt that perhaps I was adding to a problem, I should stop. The Hippocratic oath, before it was mistranslated by a monk centuries ago, was "*at least*, do no harm." If we can look back on our lives as having been lived fully without doing any harm, is this enough? Some elderly people who are dying seem to celebrate how they have loved those close to them and regret how they were not more true to themselves. Would I have loved better and been truer to myself if I had stayed in the soup kitchen? No, I think I'd be miserable and bitter, perhaps doling out a pinch of subtle meanness with every ladleful, infecting the downtrodden with an even more vicious disease than they would be exposed to while sleeping on the street.

The loss or absence of beliefs that are tied to reality can be devastating: Germany during the rise of Hitler; Jonestown; teenagers who mass murder; Afghanistan after decades of political and military conflict and economic failure. Our beliefs are the psychological counterparts to our genes; they determine the meaning of all that we do, see, and think, and are essential to our survival. People will defend their principal beliefs as strongly as they will their parents and their children, because these beliefs determine the psychological world in which they live. The loss of fundamental beliefs is associated with clinical depression, alcoholism, death, and suicide. The belief systems of elderly people may determine whether they will soon die: Those who have no faith, who question "why me?" when they fall ill, are 25 percent more likely to die within the next year than those who can place their illness in the context of their beliefs.

Everyone is vulnerable to losing their fundamental beliefs. According to her diaries, even Mother Teresa sometimes felt rejected by God, helpless, and was tempted to abandon her work caring for the poor and dying. Her struggle was life long, and her experience ranged from joy and yearning for God to doubts of God's existence. At times, she longed to leave India and return to the "beautiful things and comforts" in Europe and the "people they mix with." On occasion, her darkness even limited her ability to pray. Yet, somehow, she was able always to return to find meaning in the grace that she embodied. Her capacity to return has benefited the lives of millions of people.

It seems that, when some people fall into the dark pit of meaninglessness, they grab onto whatever will pull them out, no matter how horrible the consequences. The feeling seems to be that anything is better than nothing. Embedded in our human biology is a single governing principle: We will not stay down. We will keep coming to the surface to find the light. And, when the world is eclipsed to us, we will burrow and drive toward the most immediate point of light. If this point of light leads nowhere, we will drive and burrow toward another, and another, until the points of light become so tiny that we cannot distinguish them from the random illusive pattern on our retinas in the darkness.

When I awake from my dreams of being chased, I search for the meaning of my quest, attempting to distinguish light from illusion. This process of searching for meaning in our darkest hours helps shape the course of our lives. When we are spiritually and emotionally drowning, it determines the shore upon which we will wash, whether the island of self-protection or a new land of self-determination and serenity.

Searching for Meaning;
Finding Fear and Loathing

IN ANY HIGHER ANIMAL, the brain is primed to perceive threatening stimuli. Like children confronted with shadows, we are generally afraid of what we don't understand. The neural connections between the regions of the brain that are associated with perceiving threat and eliciting fear-generated responses are short and fast, even in humans. These neural connections are so basic and primitive in humans that they are believed to be able to act on their own, without any involvement of higher cognitive functions, like language. We have the hardwired capacity to respond fearfully without even knowing what frightens us. A series of laboratory experiments has demonstrated that fearful stimuli—pictures of snakes, disfigured humans, guns aimed at the viewer—elicit fear responses even if the stimuli are presented so quickly that the subjects aren't aware of what they're seeing. Some subjects in these experiments demonstrated physiological fear responses, such as the galvanic skin response described in the studies Roland discussed with me in chapter 3, even though they denied experiencing fear. Thus, the perception of threat and our response may completely bypass awareness, even if they're manifested in our behavior. In everyday life, this means that many people may become afraid for what seems to them to be no reason. Their fear response is aroused, and then they're either dumbfounded or they try to figure out what frightened them. Sometimes, they find the threatening stimulus; other times, they either don't find it or they're wrong about what it is.

In modern Western society, there is much that most of us don't understand, and much that is potentially frightening. Danger can seem to be everywhere at times. We often get so much information that the information itself endangers us: For example, modern medicine tries to reduce liability by informing patients of every potential harmful aspect of a treatment but, when we are told all of the details about a medical condition and its treatment, the placebo effect can be eliminated, which minimizes healing, since the placebo effect is the most powerful element of any treatment. If we believe in our doctor, we heal better and faster, yet managed care and litigation-sensitive physicians have all but eliminated the doctor-patient relationship that, in earlier days, promoted such healing. The bits of degraded knowledge we receive don't really improve our understanding; they merely give us more fodder for our fear. So, we curse the doctors, and we curse the lawyers, and we curse the legal system that allowed such destructive litigation. Yet, the fundamental component of the problem is that we, like our jury of peers, are unable to understand the information that is given to us, so we rely upon an ancient neurological circuit by responding to threat with fear. This does not heal us.

The mismanagement of fear is not restricted to the medical and legal systems. As our sources of information have become broader, more immediately available, and even unaccountable, as through the Internet, our fears have increased. There are many things to be afraid of, yet many of these dangers are very small; the fear itself is probably what's most dangerous. Our response to fear is reflected in the development of children's playgrounds over the past few decades. The playgrounds of the 1950s were made of asphalt and steel, leading to many injuries, some of them serious. Yet when fear of injury changed the emphasis in playground construction to safety, the playgrounds of the 1970s were so boring that children stopped using them. This lack of exercise was a greater health hazard than the injuries that had caused so much fear in the first place. In addition, reduced play not only is hazardous to a child's physical health, it severely disrupts essential aspects of his development. The worst part of our fears is that they can beget a worse outcome than that which inspired them.

At times, I've been frightened by what appears to be the nothingness of my life. I go soul-searching, and return empty-handed. My world, illuminated by a single candle, is forever vulnerable to this breeze that may come up, and at times my light begins to flicker, and all I can see is faltering and sputtering.

It happened again today. I can only see failure. Nothing reasonable is solace for me now. Every study that I've completed seems worthless; if not, then it's only a drop in an ocean filled with other barely interpretable findings. Each of my studies has a significant flaw. If Roland Perlmutter was like Edison, I am the anti-Edison. They saw failure as necessary steps along a path, and this path was the point of the mission; I am focused on results only and, in review, my results are naught. Like all those songs say, rain would bring me company in my misery, but I am too self-consumed to long for it. I run; I work out. Now my anger is muted and my frustration is distracted by exhaustion, but a part of my brain still feels it. Alcoholics would drink now; I am thankful that I did not inherit that gene. I hear someone use the term *middle-aged*. I am forty-three. I wonder how many days I have left.

The power of optimism arises: Perhaps these failures are a protracted drumroll droning toward the loud cymbal crash of a scientific breakthrough. I don't know. The drum is droning and I am plodding and, somewhere, a finger twitches on a trigger.

I have another recurrent dream. I have it only when I've been away from golf or from athletic activity for a month or two. In the dream, I am playing golf inside a house, and I'm struggling with two prime issues: One, I am struggling to tee up the ball by sticking my tee into the hardwood floor; two, I am trying to negotiate a shot through a doorway or window with furniture in my back swing. And as John Updike has mentioned, I am behaving as though these challenges are normal. Freudians would, of course, love my struggle with my tee: *Ja, perhaps zee golfer not only has a tee-sized schtupper, but also has great difficulty finding a schtuppee!* All of that may be true, but I do not think that is the main point of the dream. I think we have a basic need to be outside in the wild, even the fabricated wild of a golf course, manipulating tools against nature, developing our mastery with and against our fellow humans: golf, hunting, hockey, football, baseball, chasing a woolly mammoth into a ravine. When I haven't had any of this for awhile, my brain creates it for me.

Humans have been involved in intense physical activity for millions of years, and our genes developed in this environment. When we sit all day in the fluorescent light, our basic nature feels confined, even endangered; jumping into an SUV and running over a few curbs doesn't quite fill this void, so we look for activities to allow these genetically engineered drives to express themselves. War fills this need very well. Fortunately for the human race, it is not the only option. We can work symbolically. Sport can enable us to develop and exercise our warrior mentality without taking casualties, encouraging us to engage and confront our opponents and our fears.

To many of those who don't golf or do so only casually, the analogy of golfers to warriors is ridiculous. However, usually the times that a warrior is engaged in battle are few, if any, and, if few, brief. Most of the time, the warrior lives in the plateau between the rises of battle. As cadets learn at the United States Military Academy, it is important for us to engage with the activities of the plateau, since most of our lives are spent there. In addition, they are presumably the purpose of the war, no? To enable the rest of us to have the freedom to speak our minds and pursue our passions?

Golf is in part an exercise in overcoming our natural tendencies toward fear. There may have been many times that a player has hit a horrible shot with a particular club, yet focusing only on these memories and the fear they engender will lead to hesitation. Seeing negative possibilities in the perspective of a broader spectrum is the key to maneuvering through the delicate balance of risks and rewards that golf presents us. I have seen tremendous athletes become almost incapacitated by the fear of not reaching the goals that were so important to them. While this seems difficult to understand from the cozy comfort of the couch, many athletes have difficulty engaging with a task when the result is so important that a loss would be devastating. Golf provides us with repeated situations in which we must return to the task in front of us, despite the dangers of engagement. If we play golf only casually, and don't care about the dangers, then the mental exercise of golf will be as fruitful as going to the weight room to lift imaginary weights. But if we see these situations as challenges, and take them seriously, we will learn from them.

History of the Grip

THE BIGGEST FEAR that many people have is death—of ourselves and those we love. One of our greatest adaptations as a species is that we are so aware of our death that we plan for it and go to great pains to avoid it. Roland Perlmutter may have said that the frontal cortex is the part of the body that has most kept us from avoiding death, but the hand is probably a close second.

We have fifty-four bones in our hands, over 25 percent of the 206 bones in our entire body. This matrix of tiny bones is swaddled by a complex network of muscles, ligaments, and nerves that generates a vast array of forces and torques. Only primates, like us and our ape and monkey cousins, are blessed with such complicated and efficient mechanisms at the end of our wrists and, of all the primates, humans' are the most elegant. What other mechanism in the world can be employed for activities as disparate as pressing the keys on the piano to recreate Tchaikovsky, splitting a cord of wood, stroking the wisps on a baby's head, and pulling a trigger on a handgun?

For tens of thousands of years, humans have used their hands to grasp tools. Human use of tools is likely the most significant development in the history of life on earth since the first amino acid acquired the capacity to replicate itself. Perhaps nothing else is more responsible for the explosion of human population on the planet than our ability to use tools to conquer the dangers of our environment. Our evolutionary predecessors set the stage for our tool use, as they were arboreal—90 percent of their time was spent in trees, moving by grasping tree limbs and vines. Gripping was not only a matter of survival, it was the most essential element of generating motion. Deep in the caverns of our neural history is an ability to grip, grab, and hold on for dear life. Grip to go. Grip to stop. Grip to get food. Grip as tightly as possible to prevent falling to the ground and certain death.

Grip the club. It is the first lesson for any golfer. Vardon, interlocking, baseball, cross-handed, claw. How we place our hands on the club determines how we will feel our swing and how it will be initiated. Harvey Penick used to state that, if someone has a poor grip, he doesn't want a good swing, because it will be impossible to hit the ball straight. Anyone who has ever changed his grip knows how awkward the slightest change can feel before it's been fully engrained. Each finger has a specific place and function, even if, for some fingers, we are often unaware of what that place and function should be.

As told by Davis Love III in his book *Every Shot I Take*, Jimmy Hodges, a protégé of his father's, would tell his students to grip the club very firmly and waggle it, making it feel very light but uncontrollable. Then, he would have them gradually lessen the grip strength until they were barely holding on to it, making the clubhead feel like a sack of potatoes. In between these, a student could find the proper firmness that personally resonated with his swing. Harvey Penick taught that the hands should be joined as one unit, feeling as though they are melted together: "As for grip pressure, keep it light. Arnold Palmer likes to grip the club tightly, but you are not Arnold Palmer."

An important fundamental of the golf grip is the development of an awareness of grip pressure. One evening, before the Sunday of a major tournament, Jack Nicklaus ran into Greg Norman at a restaurant. Norman was in contention the next day, and Nicklaus was not, so Nicklaus offered some of the sage advice that had won eighteen major tournaments: "Monitor your grip pressure." Nicklaus felt that this was the most important aspect of allowing Norman's great talent to express itself: He needed to beware of the tendency to increase the pressure of the grip when anxiety increases.

Most golf instructors teach their players to focus on the large muscles in the body when swinging the club; beginners focus on their arms and hands, and lose clubhead speed as a result. It's natural for us to think that we should focus on the movement of our hands when swinging the club, but it is our unconscious overemphasis on our hands that interferes with the natural power of the golf swing. Many golfers completely regrip the club at the top of their swing and are never even aware of it. They vehemently deny such an absurd observation, even when it comes from a respected pro! Dick Coop did unpublished research on golfers on the UNC golf team (including Davis Love III and Jack Nicklaus, Jr.), and found that those who had increases or decreases in tension during the stroke were inferior putters. The best putters among them were those who had a *consistent* grip pressure through the putting motion. Awareness of the vicissitudes of the grip seems to be an important element of excellence in golf.

One of the ironies of teaching golfers how to monitor their grip pressure is that teachers often use images that provoke anxiety, thus causing unconscious increases in grip pressure. We have a natural tendency to respond to anxiety with movement: A seated speaker becomes emotional, then springs to his feet, and maybe even wrings his hands. We ready ourselves for danger this way. Even though we no longer live in the trees, we continue to ready ourselves for danger by preparing to grab something. Davis Love Jr. said to his son, "A grip should be like a good, firm handshake. Not so hard as to hurt somebody's fingers, but not so light that it's like shaking hands with a dead fish either." Sam Snead's quote about the grip may be the most frequently cited: He stated that the firmness of the grip should be like "holding a little bird in your hands." While Harvey Penick thought this was why Snead had no calluses on his hands, it has created calluses for a lot of other golfers. The images of squeezing a little bird to death or shaking hands with a cold fish are not exactly soothing. A golfer once noted to me that his instructor told him that the image he should have of the grip is of shaking hands with him, yet the instructor had such a clammy handshake that the golfer became squeamish every time he thought of it, and he had to struggle to erase the image from his mind. Images of grip pressure have to be associated with relaxation and calm, and are best chosen by the individual golfer, even if they make no sense to other people. One golfer I worked with used as an image for proper grip pressure a leaf that had been lying on the range next to him when he reached a very comfortable amount of firmness in his grip and began hitting the ball unusually well; he used the image of the leaf to remind himself to maintain that relaxed grip and "leaf it alone."

When I think back to the day I hit those successive drives off of the telephone pole, I recall the club feeling like an extension of my hands. I could feel where the club met my fingers and palm, but they did not feel separate. The club on my fingers felt like an additional joint I had acquired, like a knee or elbow. It was as though it were not just my driver that hovered behind the ball, but a part of me. Pilots who fly huge commercial airliners report that, despite the massive size of the vehicle at their command, they feel as though it is an extension of themselves; they feel the wings spreading out of their back, and feel the wheels on the tarmac as though they were springing out from the seat of their pants. It was the same with my driver that day. My grip on the club was where my body surface met with the external world, but it did not feel this way. It felt like I was meeting the ball with a part of myself, and the fact that the club moved of its own accord did not diminish the feeling that it was a part of me. Rather than feel as though I needed to be responsible for a series of complex angles to deliver the most accurate blow to the ball, I felt only that I needed to allow this one extension of myself to move on its own. The boundary between myself and my club, represented by my hands upon the grip of the club, had dissolved.

The intensity of my focus on the current moment helped my grip pressure. Normally, my grip on the club is very tight but, that day, it was more relaxed, more flexible, which promoted greater distance and accuracy. Since I had no responsibility for the initiation of the swing, I was not anxious about the outcome that would result. I was absorbed in the creation of the shot. There was no future, no past. No haunting failures. No prospect of looming death. This is why we normally have such trouble monitoring our grip pressure: Deep in our neural history, lying there since we were arboreal primates swinging on vines, is a natural and sudden tendency to respond to any threat to our survival by grasping onto something. Even if we are not aware that we see the danger, we tighten our grip because we are afraid to die.

Death

OUR FEAR OF DEATH is natural. Until very, very recently in historical terms, the world has been a dangerous place for human beings. For millions of years, we have been prey for other animals large and small, from ferocious beasts to opportunistic bacteria. Until the late 1700s, the average life span of a human being was approximately twenty to thirty years; the infant mortality rate was about 20 percent, and another 30 percent died before they reached five years of age.

For those who were able to stay alive, observing death was common. Anyone with a frontal cortex knew that death was inevitable, yet temporarily avoidable. Our biological and social structures seek desperately to avoid death, a brilliant mechanism to extend life and promulgate the species. This mechanism helps us protect our bodies, fight for resources, and destroy what threatens us. It has been highly successful. As a species, we are like the nerd who comes back to his high-school reunion having made a billion dollars in his computer company. Nobody pushes us around anymore. According to the U.S. Census, the average life span in the United States has grown from about thirty in 1800 to forty-nine in 1900 to seventy-seven in 2000. We have learned to stay alive. Yet, like the billionaire nerd who still flinches when he hears the word *wedgie*, we have embedded in us a physiological response to any warning signs of potential death.

You may feel that I overestimate the importance of death, but who has not wondered about the shape of his own future eulogy? Death is not just the horrid experience of dying, but the knowledge that your life is over, that your history ends at that moment. We often convince ourselves that our victories and achievements will help us to live on after we're gone. Most researchers believe their work will be cited after they've died, though only about 1 percent are ever worthy of this posthumous acknowledgement. We put our lives in high gear to outrun the reaper, deluded that our works will mount a defense against his scythe.

A friend of mine thinks often about his own death. Every little bump is a potential cancer, every raise in his heart beat is an imminent heart attack. When is it going to happen? How is it going to happen? What will be his last words? Will his wife and children mourn him? Will they be able to move on with their lives? What will his funeral be like? Will his co-workers attend, even if they didn't know him very well? Maybe he should get a little more exercise, but how much is too much? Oh no, another bad air-quality day; he'll try to breathe less deeply. He wonders if bottled water is really better, after all, it isn't tested nearly as much as municipal water—but who knows what's in *that*?

My friend's torment is but an exaggeration of what many of us experience. Some of our concerns with death have become obsolete, yet we're bred to escape death, and we love to do so. The popularity of action films is explained by viewers' identification with the hero who repeatedly escapes certain death. After watching professional wrestling on television, adolescent boys and young men videotape themselves performing the same acts, except they do the real thing: They hit each other with wooden boards and drive tacks into each other's skulls. They enjoy this. How could that possibly be? They have no immediate life-or-death struggle in which to participate, so they invent one.

I am appalled by this type of behavior, of course, though I'm really no different. The other day I was racing down a winding country road at eighty miles per hour. I don't usually get thrilled by driving a car, but I was in a hurry. After all, I had a very important . . . *appointment for a haircut!* When I finally accessed my observing ego, and asked myself why I was allowing such an insignificant part of my life to endanger the whole thing, this refrain was playing in my head: "I want to play! I want to fight! I want to play! I want to fight! I want to play!" Repeat forever. Sometimes we keep gunning the engine so that it won't stall, ready to sprint even if the starting flag is never waved.

Facing the Moment

AS OUR DRIVE TO FIGHT AND PLAY outlives its biological usefulness, it can lead to a dark rage against the waning of our youth. Yet, if we allow it to simply fade, we may find true meaning in our lives. Somewhere in the sadness that lies between enthusiasm and desperation is truth. An old man once told me, "If you're not humble by the time you're my age, you just haven't been paying attention." There is a stillness here, where we can see ourselves and others more clearly.

My six-year-old son was a participant in an experiment at the Duke Children's Hospital. His daunting task was to use a rope to swing onto a set of soft stairs, then climb up them to a swinging platform, walk across the platform, then climb onto a swinging log covered by a mat, crawl across it to a large upside-down oil drum, then sit on the drum while he took a magnetic fishing pole and fished for paper fish with metal paper clips on them. Then, he was to carry the fish back across the series of obstacles, clip it onto a clothes pin above the platform swing, crawl down the stairs, take a plastic coin from a pile, and insert it into a play cash register. Finally, he was to go to a blackboard and record how many times he completed the obstacle course. He struggled on the swinging log, and twice fell off; his immediate response was to laugh and to get the experimenter and his mother to laugh with him. He had immediately shifted from engagement in the task to a silliness about failing at the task. Then, his performance quickly worsened and he lost track of what he was supposed to do next, often forgetting to do things that he had remembered the very first time. He had lost his focus on what he was doing, and his attention had become internal. I don't know what was going on inside him; maybe he was sad or suffering or oblivious. He seemed to get angry. His interaction with the cash register changed from a sweet "change, please" to a demanding "give me some ice cream!" Anger born of distraction born of self-doubt born of failure. And I, the old block from which the chip was cut, had trouble staying with the whole scene. I had started the day tired and sad to begin with, but his struggles and primitive attempts to recover his self-esteem pierced my chest. A vision of a naked young woman from my past, sexually posed, came to mind, and I had trouble shaking it. The sexual image was so much more appealing than the twin towers of my empathy for my son's struggles and my own self-pity. My son was in the midst of responding to his failure by becoming silly, then angry; I, much the same, responded to the pain of the current moment with an unrealistic longing for a time of youthful vigor and prowess, devoid of responsibility, sex before love enriches it with future. I was like someone who nods off while hungry, and dreams that he is eating something. When he raises the dream food to his mouth and bites, he awakens to find there is nothing there!

It wasn't until the next day that I fully recovered. It was hard work. I think it would have been easier just to give in and hire a mistress, though the rewards would have been fleeting and ambivalent. Instead, I came to see the beauty of his struggle, the grace of the dance between his actions and his psyche. When he fails, he becomes distracted, silly, and angry; thoughts become more appealing than the task at hand. Me, too. We would deal with this. This was the meat and potatoes of my life, the thick substance that can bring meaning and value. My vision of the naked young woman was thin and valueless, like a brief memory of the saccharine in this morning's coffee. When I saw him after work the next day, he ran toward me with unusual exuberance and jumped into my arms. Later, when he was slow to get ready for bed, my usual impatience was infused with an emerging kindness.

~

WHEN I AM ON THE GOLF COURSE, I am no more and no less than who I am. Every shot confirms this and, if I need to learn the lesson again, golf will give it to me. If I hit a poor approach shot into a bunker, yet focus on how much I wanted to have hit it close to the pin, my regret over the past will sour the sand shot as well. Only if I accept my place in the bunker, submit fully to what is true, and focus on the shot in front of me in the present, will I be able to blast out of the sand as I intend to. After thousands of trials and errors, I have learned that I always need to be with the current shot, not the previous one or the one coming up. If I need to lay up to a certain position to attempt a difficult shot over water, and I dwell on my dread about the upcoming shot, I will certainly botch my layup. The process of learning to stay focused on the present has been extraordinarily difficult, and at times seemed impossible. Occasionally, the game presents challenges that need to be met; at those times, my eagerness becomes almost overwhelming. I can feel the excitement and anticipation in my chest and belly, and it seems like I need to breathe slowly and calmly to keep from hyperventilating. When I fail to take advantage of the opportunity, my regret is unfathomable. The walk to my next shot feels like a death march and, at times, I can literally hear

Mozart's funeral knell in the back of my mind. The most difficult part of golf is the process of emerging from this darkness, and I have often failed miserably. Yet, when I've been able to conquer this transient psychotic depression, I feel complete, needing no changes or improvements.

A nonscientific study, written by a nongolfer, reported that 99 percent of golfers' spouses were glad their spouse played golf, and that they were even more sexually satisfied than nongolfers' spouses. When I can play golf and devote myself to it, my life outside golf feels more fulfilling and important, and I'm able to give all of myself to whatever I'm doing, whether it's interacting with my wife, taking care of my children, or going to the dry cleaner. I don't know if this is because I've satisfied myself by playing golf, which allows me to be more giving, or if playing good golf requires me to be fully absorbed in what I'm doing, and this state of mind persists away from the course as well.

I remember a round of golf that I played with friends in the remnants of Hurricane Bertha. Autumn in the Raleigh-Durham area is hurricane season and, even when the hurricanes don't rip over us full force, the sporadically subtropical sky can grow turbulent, and we get some huge rainstorms that are hurricanes weakened by the 120 or so miles of land between us and the coast. Although I don't normally play golf in hurricanes (who could resist playing in a hurricane named after the most popular driver at the time?), I responded to the peer pressure to at least show up to cancel together. I was joining a group including Bob Stanger, the local amateur hero and reigning North Carolina mid-amateur champion, and didn't want to be accused of being too gutless to be a part of the group. When I arrived at the pro shop that day, and asked if the course was open, I received an unenthusiastic "yeah" from the assistant pro, which came along with an eye roll and a twisted eyebrow, free of charge. "What are the chances that Stanger will show?" I asked, apparently hoping to further the humiliating nature of this exchange. The pro accommodated me by silently thrusting in my face his fingers in the shape of a zero. I think his answer also reflected what he thought of me. I headed out to the first tee anyway, and was joined by another desperado. As soon as we teed off, Bob came trotting up, hit, and off we went.

Playing golf in a hard rain always reminds me of running a small business. Not only do I need to hit the next shot with a wet grip, a slippery stance, and a flyer lie, but I have to manage my umbrella against the wind, keep my towels off the ground, and try to keep something, anything, on me dry. The tendency is to speed up, to hurry down the fairway to the next shot, as though you'll be ducking into a building when you get to your ball. Except the building never comes. I double-bogeyed the first hole, taking four hurried, wet, thoughtless whacks at the ball across a rivulet-infested fairway before reaching a soaked but playable first green. I wasn't even very upset about my score, given the circumstances. Yet, I was visited by the consciousness I have when I awake from my running-terrified-away-from-natives nightmare: "What am I doing playing here?" It was an easy question to ask. One of the assistant pros had even said, "Why aren't you home with your family?" I had first thought that he was jealous, since I got to play and he was stuck folding shirts all day, but then I started to wonder if he was right. What were we doing in this hurricane remnant scurrying around like a murder of crows in a cornfield? I suddenly longed for my wife and my children, and cursed myself for being out there.

I have never read any research on the relationship between sadness and performance in golf, but I have always played better when I'm sad. I don't really know why. As I mentioned earlier, there is a wealth of data suggesting that people who are mildly depressed make more realistic judgments of themselves: Ask a group of depressed people and a group of nondepressed people to perform a little task, like playing a number-guessing game, and then ask them all how they did; the nondepressed people will think they did better than they actually did, while the depressed people, especially those who are only mildly depressed, will assess their performance accurately. They are better at seeing themselves for who they are.

Theory holds that they're depressed because they see through to their limitations, their warts and all. However, the opposite arrow of causality seems to apply as well: To surface from their sadness, people who are mildly depressed need to take a clearer look at themselves so they can develop a plan to improve their circumstances. Maybe when I'm sad, I am more accepting of who I am; I'm not fleeing myself by creating lofty notions of who I will be. I am with myself, with all of my faults and weaknesses. When Phil Mickelson won the Buick Invitational at Torrey Pines in 2001 after having had serious food poisoning, he said that he sometimes plays better when he's sick because he is "too weak to have expectations." That day, I felt my weaknesses to the point that I had no expectations at all. Also, I felt the emptiness of some of the things that drove me to golf so much: lowering my handicap, preparing for a local tournament, beating my friends in our weekly match. I didn't even have to grab myself by the collar and force my nose into the accident I had just left on the carpet by asking, "What about the starving people in Africa?" There were people starving for my attention in my own home, and I missed them. Somehow, this sadness and longing allowed me to dismiss my investment in whether this "small business" I was operating on the course was successful. Released from the burden of this usual expectation, I was able to bring my full focus to the current shot. And, in the current shot, I found the answers to the questions that were spinning through my mind. The richness of the task in front of me was powerful and meaningful in itself. I loved the shot. I did. I do.

Playing in the downpour only enhanced the usual primitive

struggle. I was reminded of a rock outcropping I had seen along a turbulent Puerto Rican shore, visible only after a wave receded: For centuries, it had been pounded by the surf, yet still it protruded into the chaotic and violent world around it. I strongly felt the need to be out on the course, facing a challenge from nature, from other people, and from my own physical limitations. The elemental nature of this activity was meaningful in itself, as itself, and the comic circumstances only supported the basic meaning I had felt. I am afraid of how trite this may sound, but I feel that it's true: My family, dry at home, missed me that day; yet, with each shot, I became for us a better man.

If not for this transition from a focus on the result at all costs to a focus on the process, golf is indeed a meaningless game. Like Edison's process of discovery, each failure and success is a necessary step of learning along the journey of the task. *This filament doesn't light when it's charged with such a current. Fascinating. I'll try another.* The main point is not that while golf seems meaningless to the outside observer, it is in fact full of meaning; the point is that golf *is* meaningless, yet it's still an exercise in understanding how to join with the process of who we are, where we are, and what challenges stand before us. This is not part of the meaning of golf; it is the only meaning in golf, unless you think all those numbers really mean something, or there's inherent value in the act of striking a ball with a stick. Only when we dismiss the illusions of meaning can we stare into the void that remains; only then, can the richness of the moment spring forth.

One natural self-criticism, a remnant of the self-loathing, is that this interpretation of the nothingness of golf is merely a justification for comfort. It is much easier to swallow our luxury if we can rationalize that it has some greater cosmic purpose. How do we know if the purpose generated from this view of nothingness is good? In response to a monk who became consumed with the idea of having a particular possession, St. Francis of Assisi, quoting Jesus, said to him: "A man possesses in learning only so much as comes out of him in action, and a monk is a good preacher only so far as his deeds proclaim him as such, for a tree is known by its fruits." What are the fruits of the labors of our love of golf and sport? Does the view of the nothingness in them engender hatred or kindness? Does it lead to hoarding or generosity? Does it lead us to inspire others to live in terror or freedom? We all answer these questions differently but, by the answers, do we know the worth of our passion.

~

LIVING IN NEW YORK CITY for several years, then moving to North Carolina's version of a turbocharged prefabricated development in Cary (considered by locals an acronym meaning Containment Area for Relocated Yankees), it was difficult to imagine that the world's population growth is slowing. In the Containment Area, many of the rivers ran reddish brown with the silt of the local clay that had been dug up by home builders and developers. Farms were bulldozed and replaced with shopping centers and parking lots with bizarrely shaped mazelike patterns of accessibility to prevent drivers from using them as shortcuts. Forests were leveled for cul-de-sacs with English-sounding names like Wittenham Court. One community near a tennis facility chose to name its streets after famous tennis players; since 1989, there has been an Agassi Court. (Can you imagine living on a street named for a then-petulant nineteen-year-old?) The dramatic change that has occurred on the planet was brought to the fore one day when our next-door neighbor's son found a Confederate coin sticking out of the soil in his backyard. Less than 150 years ago, in this triangle of computers and biotechnology, men had paused to rest and allow their horses to drink from the stream that lines the edge of the property. They were tired, for they had been preparing to kill or die to prevent the North from telling them how to live their lives and whom they could own. Today, the dangers are not so stark, but hidden, almost subterranean. Arthur C. Clarke envisioned that the year 2001 would be marked by discoveries in space, and cold, emotionless interactions with computers and each other. Everyone in my little cul-de-sac worked for IBM and, at times, it seemed to me that their voices sounded like Clarke's computer HAL as it was being turned off by an astronaut: programmed to appear calm, yet distant and scared as hell. Our lawns were neat and the children were clean, but there was an anguish below the surface that I could not name. Or maybe it was me: Sometimes I long for the grit and the grime from which we sprung.

Mystical experience is often depicted with images of heavenly light raining on a subject from above, or the twinkling of auras around his or her soul. In reality, it's much grittier than that. Whether on the golf course or in the church, mystical experience is characterized by a dramatic shift in attention to the richness of the present. The hands of the mystic are not always clean; they are covered with the earthiness of the moment, and the mystic feels his hands fully, whether they're dipped in mud or dabbed with blood. The shift of attention to the current moment overwhelms other concerns. Religious belief and mystical experiences provide defections from our death-survival bubble and its anxious vapors by allowing us to stay focused on the present.

All religions have ways of contending with death. The major religions seem to diminish the importance of this life through reference to the next one, whether the next life is an ongoing series as in the reincarnation of Hinduism and Buddhism, or the single evaluated opportunity of Christianity, Judaism, and Islam. All these approaches effectively reduce our daily concerns with dying: If this life is but one in a series, losing it is not so awful; if it's a mere test for where we will spend eternity, we had better increase our intensity about what we're doing now, instead of worrying about when the test will end. The prospect of returning to God at the end of this life is particularly reassuring, and greatly diminishes the fear of death for many.

From a scientific perspective, many of these religious views have an accurate basis. Regarding the Eastern notion of reincarnation, our genes have been passed to us through thousands of generations, and they will continue to be refined and perfected, depending upon chance and the environment of the future, although science makes no claims about what the end of the story will be; Nirvana and heaven on earth are only calculable probabilities. The Western idea of returning to God after death seems true even from the view of psychology: When we live, we touch a multitude of other lives, and, when we're gone, the memory of us lives in them, affects them, saddens them, encourages them, inspires them, or, perhaps, serves as an example of how not to be. What others have gathered from us is passed on through the generations. I live and breathe not only with my father's genes, but with the lessons his world gave him. After our death, our life—our work—becomes a part of the vast human community and the nature that surrounds it. We become one with everything. We return to the largeness and greatness of God.

Golf is fraught with symbolic death and, in response to it, we often become anxious and ready to grab. Since there are no vines to hold onto, our grip gets tighter, and we lose power in our drives and roll our wrists over our three-footers. The image of failure on the course triggers a primitive fear response. The elimination of this primitive response is the crowning glory of a good round. It is also the full expression of our phylogenetic distance from other species. We are able mentally to move beyond our natural tendency to grow tense in the face of danger; we can be conscious of our imminent death, yet face it without fear. It seems to me sometimes that, more than anything else, this is why we love golf: It enables us, it *demands* of us, to stand strong and calm against our primitive fears and urges.

While these moments of calm and absorption in the present are tremendously rewarding in themselves, they are often followed by an even more powerful experience. A golfer who no longer needs to try to become focused on the present, but who actually *is* focused on the present, becomes available to those around him. When our attention to our individual struggles on the golf course is weakened, we can shift our view toward the struggles of others. Most everyone has felt this at one time or another: You suddenly realize that not only is your golf performance acceptable, but that you're outside in pleasingly sculpted nature with people you care about and, perhaps, even enjoy. This experience is a brief sniff of the transformation that occurs in people who have had mystical experiences. When the self is temporarily obliterated, engrossment with others rushes in with the thundercrack of air filling the vacuum produced by lightning.

Many saints have devoted their lives to caring for other people after a single experience of mystical union with God. The certainty of their everlasting communion with God enabled them to abandon their individual, selfish quests, and turn toward nurturing the growth of other people. A Buddhist *bodhisattva* is someone who stands at the doorway to the immortality of nirvana, having spent his whole life in pursuit of enlightenment yet, at the last moment, turns around to see the suffering of others behind him, and heads back to help bring them along the path he has negotiated. As exemplified in the extreme by saints and bodhisattvas, a legitimate concern for others results not from constraint, but from a diminished regard for our own death. These experiences are glimpses of human potential: Those who have them may be the first pilgrims of our next evolution, moving beyond death by bringing the fullness of life to others.

Human concerns for the self and the community are often in conflict. Almost all political struggles, such as the juxtaposition of capitalism and socialism, reflect the balance of these two concerns. Working in combination, however, the two have helped us to reach such wondrous achievements as the dramatic increase in our life expectancy. Some species in nature, such as slime molds, act more directly as individuals and communities at the same time. Slime molds spend most of their lives as separate single-celled amoebalike organisms but, upon the release of a chemical signal, the individual cells aggregate into a great swarm of up to 100,000 cells, one large bag of cytoplasm with many nuclei. When facing unfavorable conditions, such as a local scarcity of water or food, the aggregate rises to form a tower in a matter of hours. The tip of the tower then bursts into the air, allowing individual spores to ride on air currents to greener pastures. This cycle of individual and community behavior lets the species find the best conditions to survive and thrive.

Are humans developing the same capability? As we learn to connect with each other across the planet, from the printing press to the jet airplane to the Internet, are we beginning to serve the greater whole like the aggregated cells of a slime mold? If so, might these experiences of genuine concern for others, whether by mystics or athletes, preview a future in which the members of our species begin to act in concert? When we move beyond our concerns for personal death, and the many anxieties it spawns, we gravitate toward concern about the welfare of others, whether this concern is directed toward the entire species, the entire planet, or the community in which we live. Are mystical experiences the seeds of this movement?

We have great difficulty trusting ourselves. We've been raised to keep guardrails along the sides of the highway of our lives; we imagine that any small deviation from the straight and narrow will send us hurtling off a precipice. Trusting one's self can be frightening, since we all have thoughts and impulses we don't want to follow. How will we be able to stop ourselves from following immoral, or even insane or illegal, impulses once we start to pry the fingers of restraint from around our hearts? We are not only afraid of death and failure but, also, of being too successful, too powerful, of being the malevolent dictators that we would have become had our parents and teachers not intervened. This mistrust of our inner nature creeps into every aspect of our lives, including our tendency to hold fast to our traditions, our laws, and, even, our thoughts. To think in a completely different way makes us vulnerable to losing what we have and who we are—and most of us have worked at those projects for a long time. To open ourselves up to new thoughts and new mental experiences is to expose ourselves to the possibility of being different, of being wrong, of becoming psychotic. We are afraid to take the chance of losing what we hold dear.

As Roland Perlmutter taught me years ago, many of these fears are unfounded; our central nervous system has developed in such a way that we know much more than we think we know. We fear that if we become absorbed in the steps we're taking, we will lose direction and drift off the path into the woods. Yet, increased awareness of the process of our life does not eliminate our sense of where we're headed, it just reduces the amount of time we spend worrying about it. As we learn to trust ourselves, we get feedback about the rightness or indecency of our path. It is by the fruits of our efforts that our efforts are judged. Our awareness has the potential gradually to blossom and be nurtured, or to be poisoned by how it's received by ourselves and others. With time and intention, our awareness learns what nurtures it and how it can grow stronger.

CHAPTER EIGHT

Spawning the
Effortless Present

I HAD ORIGINALLY INTENDED to end this book with the previous chapter. It seemed as though a description of my pursuit of understanding my experience from the perspectives of neuroscience, intuition, sport psychology, and spirituality was enough. With a mixture of hesitation and excitement, I sent the draft of my manuscript to Roland Perlmutter. I did not hear from him. While I waited, I sweated through a few weeks of fantasies of his laughing at me, interrupted by an occasional brief vision of his telling me how brilliant I am. Finally, I gave his office a call to see if he had had a chance to look it over, or perhaps to nudge him in that direction if necessary. His secretary informed me that he was over at the Duke Comprehensive Cancer Center. He was not lecturing there. He was dying.

I visited him that afternoon. I was so sad to hear of his illness that I forgot all about my book and the collaborative studies that we were planning together. He had been such a vibrant man, so fully *alive*, that, as I walked down the hallway to see him, I feared what he would look like, and how I would react to his having withered from the treatment he had received over the past two weeks. I practiced being undaunted by his frail form, trying only to see the person behind the ghostly figure I expected.

He did not appear to be nearly as ill as I had envisioned. In fact, he looked calm, and still had the same fire in his eyes that usually accompanied him during our discussions.

"Roland," I stammered as our eyes met and he sat up, smiling, happy to see me. "I had no idea . . ."

"No shit. Me, either. After all these years of studying intuition and unconscious understanding of even the most mundane brain processes, I couldn't see my own cancer spreading through me like a cold through a kindergarten. And I'm a physician!"

Roland seemed to be even less inhibited than usual, like he had had a couple of drinks or too much caffeine. I wasn't sure if this was due to his imminent death or a side effect of the medication he was getting.

"I've read a few articles about the kind of cancer I have," he continued, "and I don't stand a chance against this thing. I was really pissed for a while, but I've come to this weird calm and acceptance lately. It's really hard to explain. I'm not cursing the things I don't get to do or even the people I'll leave behind. I mean, I'll miss them and I feel very, very full of sorrow sometimes, but it doesn't feel like something I need to fight or even change. I never thought it would be this way; I always thought I'd be scared as hell and horrified of the prospect of not *being* any more, but I feel more fortunate for what I've had and who I am than anything else. This was a total surprise."

I stood and listened, grateful that he was not miserable, and less guilty for not having done something, even though there had never been anything for me to do. As usual, Roland's presence had the effect of allowing me to be fully with him and more fully with myself than I usually was. I was even able to be with his death without wanting to be somewhere else. I would normally want to run away from the social discomfort of this type of situation, but the elemental nature of how he viewed his passing left me feeling honored to be with him in the process of it.

"I've been thinking of calling you," he said. "I wasn't sure if it was because I was sick and wanted to talk with you about it, to connect about it like we do sometimes, or whether it was because of your book."

I was flattered that he, too, felt the connection between us. I realized at that moment that I had never considered that he was getting something out of our conversations, too; I had always been so enthralled with what he was giving me, it never occurred to me that he was similarly engaged. I stayed silent as he spoke again.

"I'm still not sure, but I kind of worked out this death thing on my own. I've been thinking about your book, and I don't want you to take this the wrong way . . . like I said, I've really gotten a lot out of our conversations, and I know that I did most of the talking, but you've been a tremendous listener, and I always feel like I'm really, really smart when I talk to you, and I think that helps me get to some ideas that I would not have come upon otherwise."

I swallowed hard, afraid almost to breathe. He did not hesitate.

"I think it's a shame that people rarely say what they really think about someone unless they're overcome with emotion or about to die, but it's been very important for me to let you know how I feel about these things."

"I've felt privileged to listen to you," I said, finally able to speak. "I'm hoping to hear a lot more from you," I said, but did not believe.

He confronted my hypocrisy immediately. "You won't. Don't kid yourself, and you certainly won't kid me. I have a few weeks, tops." He was no longer sad, but seemed about to launch into a mission, like a plane taxiing on a runway or a lion circling his prey. "I've wanted to talk to you about the draft of the book you sent me because I think you're selling yourself short," and he landed on the last three words with a focused deliberateness—*selling yourself short*. "And, frankly, you're selling me short. Maybe this is why I've been avoiding calling you. I knew that it would be hard for you, since I'm dying and now I'm going to tell you that you need to take the next step on this whole topic. And I probably won't be around to help you, but let me tell you a little bit about what I've been thinking.

"You've confused the foothills for the mountaintops," he said with a solemn chagrin, shaking his head. "You've learned how to attain the experience of life climbing out of you, and you see that it may be related to something bigger than all of us, but how are other people going to get farther along? You refer to it a bit at the end, but if the human race is ever to act in unison like a slime mold, how do you think this is going to happen? Through magic? It's going to take a huge effort based upon truth. Only science can be the backbone for something like this."

I stood riveted. I realized he was probably holding back to some measure, knowing how devastating his opinion could be to me. His disappointment ripped into me, while the idea that he was going to take me even further in his thinking exhilarated me. I felt stunned, and strangely afraid to move.

"You need to understand more about how the brain changes over time," he began. "I know that you know that it's possible for older people like you and me to change the way we think about things, maybe even to generate new neurons in some brain regions. But how do we take advantage of what we've learned about our own neural circuitry? It's not just an interesting fact, like the number of ants that live in a colony; it has the potential to change the course of humanity! And what if we could take this tack from the start? What if we could alter the course of how the brain develops *deliberately*, with the whole plan directed toward enabling people to experience the *effortless present*? Do you really want to just tell a little story about how you came upon this one day on a driving range, then you found out that it was sort of a brain experience and sort of a mystical experience, but that you don't really know what it is? I don't even think you really believe that!"

I was afraid of where Roland might take this. I was concerned that he would get off track, but I was probably more afraid that he had always seen into the heart of me, and that he was now going to tell me about each and every wart he saw.

He took a deep breath. I felt grateful for whatever brain process was making him temper his remarks. He had the look of a scientist again.

"Brain function changes drastically across the life span, and for good reason. What we need to learn as infants is a lot different from what we need to learn as adults. Some people suffer as adults because they never really make the switch from functioning mentally like children. Some people who seem childish are those who never really learned as children. Others are just the opposite; they learned what not to do, but they act as though their daddy is standing next to them with the switch, about to smack them for making a wrong move. You see, most of the brain activity of human infants and children is focused on inhibiting incorrect or inappropriate action."

As I listened to him, I remembered the feeling when my children were small that I was a *no* machine, spitting out instructions on what not to do like a drone broadcasting a single radio signal of denial, never allowance.

"This learning is essential, of course," he continued, "since there are so many ways to do things incorrectly, and all of the random acts of children need to be shaped into a tolerable human being. Yet, the process of learning how to behave as we develop will largely determine how we experience initiating action as adults. Will our actions come bundled with fear, or with the assumption of a warm reception from the world outside? Our ability to allow action to arise so that it seems to occur on its own is greatly affected by the emotions and the intensity of our expectations. If we focus on the specific acts that we're about to make, and not on how they'll be perceived by others, we can resolve our intentions with little additional effort."

Roland was now rolling, and I drifted over to take the lone chair in his small hospital room.

"Yes, you'd better sit down; I have a lot to tell you. And don't feel like you have to talk. I mean, you can, but I've got a few points to make, and you don't want to interrupt some of the final words of a dying man, do you?" He smirked, feigning a threatening position with his eyes. I smiled and nodded at him, indicating my willingness to be silent.

Roland began describing to me that the human child has the longest period of dependence upon caregivers of any mammal. "While the parents in most other species show their children the door by age three," Roland said, "human parents are lucky if children can care for themselves by twenty-three. One of the most important accomplishments of this seemingly endless period of time is the brain development necessary to carry out complex mental tasks, especially like developing an understanding of how people interact with each other. These accomplishments increase the likelihood that the kids will eventually become independent by ensuring success in the fundamental human activities that will ease the transition out of our hair, like getting a job.

"Some brain functions are innate, and a human would be able to do them regardless of what the environment provides. But a lot of other things the brain learns to do are dependent upon experience. In fact, much of the development of the cortex is affected by the experiences one has while growing up. Our brain is incredibly flexible—our neuronal circuits are ready to grow in just about any direction the outside world dictates. It's pretty obvious how adaptive this is. Look at the various circumstances under which humans have been able to survive: desert heat, arctic cold, drought, flood, famine, war, physical abuse, sexual abuse. The human brain has always figured a way to adapt to these situations, and grow to accommodate them, although of course it prefers things like soft touch and pleasant music over violent threats and whacks on the head.

"The dependence of certain regions of brain growth on experience is reflected in the results from some of the fMRI studies of brain activation during the recognition of letters and numbers. Functional MRI work suggests that letter recognition activates a very specific brain area. The recognition of the letters of the English alphabet is obviously dependent upon experience, since children in different cultures learn to recognize only the letters or characters in their own languages. Thus, experience determines how this highly specific brain region will develop. The brain activation that occurs when children begin to recognize letters is likely to lead to short-range activation of neighboring neurons that generates increased growth between them. As they continue to learn letters, and develop the expectation that letters will occur together to form words, the associative connection of letters with each other is strengthened. Since letters tend to be presented more frequently next to other letters than to numbers, identifying a number in a string of letters is far easier (and faster) than finding a specific letter in a string of letters. Because of the way this very specific brain region develops through very specific interactions with the environment, a number is seen against a backdrop of letters as a white object would be seen against a backdrop of blue. Only after years of experience-dependent brain growth is such an interaction possible."

I knew this, and I had read the studies he mentioned, but I knew he was setting a stage, perhaps as much for himself as for me and, since I wanted him to get up on that stage, I nodded interest, offering something I found to be surprising: encouragement. I had never had to encourage Roland before, but despite his brilliance and the almost-evangelical quality of his speech, he seemed to need it this time.

Fueled by my encouragement or by his inner drive, he marched on. "Some of the most poignant effects of the environment on brain development in infants can be found in studies of maternal touch. Infant humans and monkeys who have been deprived of contact with their mothers will have markedly impaired social abilities. If they are deprived of proper maternal care or handling, they'll develop abnormal neuronal connectivity in brain regions that are important in experiencing emotion and in the ability to send and receive social signals. This deprivation of social contact in the first few weeks of life leads to permanent neuronal changes, even if normal maternal interaction begins later. While we obviously don't do these kinds of experiments on humans, you can see the effects of experience on brain development by looking at the brain structure of people who have had different experiences. When adults listen to music, very different regions of the brain are activated in musicians than in non-musicians. The degree of activation of a brain region called the *left planum temporale* correlates strongly with the age at which a musician had begun musical training. All of this work strongly suggests that the brain reorganizes itself based upon how it has been used in the past.

"While these studies point to brain growth potential in unusual circumstances, there is also a strong role for experience in typical human brain development. It appears that much of our learning during childhood is devoted to things that are dangerous, socially inappropriate, or distressing. Most kids learn to do the right thing primarily by learning all the things that they *shouldn't* do. The early life of an infant is concerned with regulating basic biological states, such as hunger, thirst, pain and other distress. Up to about three months of age, a child can be calmed by rocking; parents later have the option of getting the infant to pay attention to something other than the distress, like a rattle or toy. However, as soon as the infant's attention returns to his internal state, the distress level rises back to what it was before. The distraction doesn't cure the distress, it just gets the infant to pay attention to something else temporarily. Developing these attentive skills will be crucial later for meeting a host of demands that life will place on the child.

"The control of emotional state and attention is regulated in part by the anterior cingulate. The eventual detailed development of this brain structure in adult humans is greatly affected by these early experiences of moving in and out of attention to distress. Children under three years of age are generally unable to inhibit their impulses. However, at about the time they turn four, they begin to develop the ability to inhibit themselves from doing what comes immediately to mind. Brain imaging studies have shown that, as a child gets older, the size of the anterior cingulate begins to determine the ability to focus attention and inhibit the impulse to pay attention to irrelevant stimuli. The extent of the development of this brain structure thus determines how well a child can shut down the impulses to do the wrong thing, and choose to activate the motor programs that will lead to the right thing.

"During childhood through adolescence, important changes occur in the brain, and it is likely that these changes differ between the gray matter and white matter of the brain. The gray exterior of the brain is generally involved in specific functions, while the interior white matter of the brain is generally associated with connections between brain regions. Crudely, the white matter of the brain connects the regions of the gray matter as a communication infrastructure of a city connects the various homes, businesses, and institutions in the city."

I was happy that I knew much of what Roland was discussing, but I felt a little alienated, in that he didn't seem to realize that we had talked about some of this before. I wasn't sure if he was going over this background because his memory was failing, or because he wanted to make sure that I had all the relevant research fresh in my mind. Maybe he knew that I would be writing this all down someday, and he wanted us to get it right, to be complete and correct in case one of his colleagues chose to question what he had said after he was gone.

Sensing the slightest retreat of my attention from him, he raised his voice slightly. "Now, this part is crucial for understanding how you can have an impact on the developing brain. You see, different parts of the brain develop at different rates, and some stop developing much earlier than others. Cortical gray matter volume increases throughout childhood and, then, in adolescence some regions continue to grow, while other growth dissipates. Volumes of the frontal and parietal lobe gray matter peak at age twelve, whereas temporal lobe volume peaks at sixteen years. Of course, the reduction in gray matter is actually a good thing, as it leads to more specificity and differentiation of functions within the brain. It's wonderful! The functions of local brain regions become more specific, and unnecessary connections between neurons are pruned away, leading to improved task performance. All the unnecessary brain connections are kind of killed off from lack of use. In contrast, the white matter continues to grow through to young adulthood. Some of these increases are limited to specific regions. For instance, the white matter in the dorsal prefrontal cortex," he pointed to where a horn might be on a cow, "increases substantially more than the white matter in the ventral prefrontal regions," as he said this he moved his fingers over to an area just above and between his eyes, motioning with his fingers that the area was deeper inside his head.

"The prefrontal cortex appears to be one of the last brain regions to mature, particularly the dorsolateral prefrontal cortex. The importance of this aspect of development for you, Rich, is that the brain regions that change the most over the course of development—that is, those that are not fully developed until late adolescence—are naturally more sensitive to environmental factors. This means that the prefrontal regions of the brain are more dependent upon experience, including adolescent experience, than any other brain region. Through adolescence, decreases in the density of gray matter neurons and increases in white matter neurons lead to a strengthening of the remaining connections. This process underlies the adage that 'neurons that fire together, wire together.' Any repeated response to the outside world will become faster, and the neural circuits that regulate that response will become stronger. The connections that underlie responses that are inhibited—usually because they are incorrect and hence get punished somehow—tend to wither. I hope you understand this, because it may be one of the most important features of human development, and more than ever we need to keep this in mind. Society has gotten so complex, and we have all these dangerous tools lying around like guns and cars, and so we need to realize that adolescents are *supposed* to make mistakes—it is a crucial part of their development. And, a lot of times, the ones who look like they are destined for lives of crime are really just in the process of learning. I know, I know, there are plenty of sociopaths who will never change but, when it comes to our kids, don't we want to err on the side of possibility? Take the kid who has a beer, then gets in a car, has an accident, and someone dies. I read about a case like this up in New York the other day. Well, whose fault is that? The kid's? The parents'? Society, for allowing kids to drive? Beer distributors? I don't know what the answer is, but I know—and this is a —ing fact, Rich—that human brain growth is structured in such a way that mistakes in judgment during adolescence are an essential component of learning in even the best and brightest among us. That's why it really chafes my tit·ends when some D.A. wants to make headlines as a Great Protector for sending some kid to jail for being unlucky."

I agreed with him, yet I worried that he was going to spiral out of control, or start frothing at the mouth. His eyes were getting wilder and more intense. I found myself nodding with more enthusiasm so that he would feel like I really understood him and that he didn't need to raise his intensity level any higher to get my attention.

"Anyway, to get back on track here, the development of concentration and memory in kids is a very tricky business. Believe it or not,

the divergent tasks of deciding to do the right thing and refrain-
ing from doing the wrong thing are regulated by largely different
brain regions. As in younger children, some of the most important
lessons that adolescents need to learn are concerned with how *not*
to do things. Substantial brain matter is devoted to these kinds
of inhibitory mechanisms, and they are very important for any
kind of social learning. A lot of childhood behavior problems, like
attention-deficit disorder, hyperactivity, and oppositional behavior,
involve symptoms that reflect an inability to *inhibit* inappropriate or
unwanted behavior.

"Studies that compare the brain activation of children and adults
while they're completing tests of attention and memory suggest that
the prefrontal cortex is activated differently in children than it is in
adults. Children have more activation of the dorsolateral prefrontal
cortex than adults during many tasks, such as trying to keep very
specific information in mind for a few seconds, or choosing whether
to respond to a series of stimuli. Yet, for this latter task, they have
less activation of the ventral prefrontal cortex than adults do. These
findings suggest that as children grow into adults, they develop a
more extensive system for *not* doing the *wrong* thing. Much of the
development of mastery and skill, then, is weeding out all the neural
connections that lead to unwanted actions. Yet the process of learning how not to make mistakes will be very different, depending upon
how the child or adolescent and the world around her interact with
each other. This process can be ripe with the development of connections to parts of the brain that experience fear, or it can be relatively streamlined, connecting only to the relevant parts of a learned
skill."

I began to see where he was taking me. The development of athletes involves learning to cope with mistakes and the fear that they
engender. Young people whose coaches teach by instilling fear
will associate the athletic moves they're supposed to learn with that
fear, and will be much more likely to have trouble performing those

moves under competitive pressure later. They will disappoint themselves and others, and will feel like chokers. Those who have learned by attending only to the move they want to make are much more likely to thrive under pressure later. These athletes are far more likely to be able to compete in the effortless present. I remembered hearing about some ongoing studies of Olympic athletes and their families that supported this contention. The intensely critical parents who drive their children out of their own frustration are actually hard to find among American medal winners, suggesting that those who thrive in the moment of athletic experience are largely competing out of an internal drive, not the horsewhip of an external motivator. I hoped that Roland would eventually get to how the brain chooses the correct moves, inhibits the incorrect moves, and how early brain development and even later adult discipline can facilitate the experience of the effortless present.

A nurse came in to take Roland's vital signs. She inserted a thermometer in his mouth for a few seconds, and he seemed like a teakettle at full boil, about to explode. His lips puckered around the plastic disposable covering of the thermometer like a child who has been told *no* too many times, which I found ironic, and I started to snicker at him. He, too, saw the irony, and gently growled at the nurse. Who knows what ideas were not being expressed during this brief interlude? And, as in a symphony, the interlude itself was pleasing, and accentuated the rhythm of Roland's cadence, which, with the beep of the thermometer indicating that the registration of Roland's temperature was complete, would now begin again.

"The first step in understanding how the brain allows the experience of the effortless present is to understand how it inhibits the many motor movements that are at its disposal, how it chooses among them, and how it monitors the results that come from them. Much of this activity is regulated by the frontal cortex, particularly the anterior cingulate."

(We have known for decades of the role of the anterior cingulate in motivating, shutting down responses, and perceiving danger. The passivity of monkeys who had this region of the brain experimentally removed led to the idea that frontal lobotomies would help to reduce the aggressiveness of violent humans, and thousands of these operations were performed in the middle decades of the twentieth century. Brain surgery to remove the anterior cingulate is still performed for people who have such severe, untreatable obsessive-compulsive disorder that they cannot stop themselves from thinking about whether they've performed certain acts properly. The anterior cingulate has long been described as being involved in *error detection*, as it becomes active when people make mistakes, and people who have had it removed seem not to care as much about the consequences of their actions. It now appears that this brain region may be involved in detecting the conditions under which errors are likely to occur rather than the actual errors themselves. It could be that when a person is confused about what move to make next because there is some conflict present in the motor system, the anterior cingulate becomes active to help draw attention to the conflict in an effort to resolve it. This is sometimes experienced as a vague sense of unease. People may say or feel that an action or a situation "just doesn't feel right." Others describe it as a *feeling of no.*)

"Let me give you a good example of what we're learning about the functioning of the anterior cingulate," he said, his enthusiasm rising a notch. Roland's use of the phrase "what we're learning" suggested that he had temporarily put aside his awareness of his imminent death; *he* was fully in the present and, as such, did not concern himself with the absence of a future.

"Research subjects in an fMRI scanner completed a test of attention that required them to press a button whenever they saw an *A* followed by an *X* in a series of letters presented at a rate of one per second. The results suggested that, while many different parts of the frontal cortex were active when errors were made, only the anterior cingulate was active in circumstances when an error was more likely, yet not made, such as when an *A* was followed by a letter other than *X*. The presence of the *A* increased the chances that they would forget to press the button if the *X* came up next, and the anterior cingulate became active even if they remembered to do so. These results suggest that the anterior cingulate monitors competition between processes that conflict during task performance."

I thought of how this might apply to someone putting. When you're trying to make a putt, having conflicting plans or information such as the grain of the grass on the green running toward the golfer putting down a slope may lead to the *feeling of no*. The golfer may translate this signal into a feeling of *there's no way I can make this putt*.

Roland continued:

"Very recent research suggests that the role of the anterior cingulate is not just to signal danger or conflict, as it's activated whenever a person pays significant attention to himself or his own performance, even if an error is no more likely. It may be that this region becomes active whenever a person has reason to look harder at himself or what he is doing. Some studies show anterior cingulate activation if a reward is not given after a correct response; this activation may indicate that the research subject is becoming motivated enough to care about how his performance is judged. People with obsessive-compulsive disorder, who often have repeated and unwanted thoughts about how others perceive them, have particularly high anterior cingulate activation when monitoring their own performance. Healthy control subjects show similar activation when they're involved in self-critical activities, such as deciding whether emotionally significant words (e.g., stingy, bold, geek) apply to them. Anterior cingulate activation also takes place when subjects take too long to decide which response to make, even if they make the correct decision. The anterior cingulate may thus become active whenever a person becomes motivated to view himself or his performance from the perspective of other people. If the anterior cingulate could speak, it would most likely say 'How am I doing?'

"This activation provides a variety of important functions: It keeps us away from doing dangerous or socially inappropriate things; it enables us to monitor our behavior continuously; it helps us maintain our motivation about our performance; and it facilitates our attention toward what we will do in the immediate future. However, if we let this activation become our *raison d'être*, it can inhibit our attention to the effortless present. The feeling of *yes*, which comes from being in the effortless present, is disrupted by the feeling of *no*, which comes with anterior cingulate activation. The extent to which the anterior cingulate is activated is the extent to which we will be hesitant, fearful, and self-conscious in our movements. One of the most interesting developments in recent research is that the anterior cingulate is active and helps us change our behavior even if we aren't fully aware that our movements have changed.

"Some recent research has demonstrated how this *feeling of no* is associated with an increase in anterior cingulate and ventral prefrontal cortex activation, as well as a reduction in the automatic performance of the effortless present. One group of researchers tested the responsiveness of the anterior cingulate and neighboring prefrontal cortex by varying the amount of time subjects needed to inhibit a response that had become overlearned and automatic. An increase in the percentage of time that subjects were given feedback that their automatic response was incorrect led subjects to have greater overall activation of the anterior cingulate and ventral prefrontal cortex prior to each response, even though the subjects were unaware that their automatic responses were less likely to be correct. So, the anterior cingulate is active not only when people become aware they are about to make an error, but it is also active when the environment changes so that the usual response becomes slightly less likely to be correct.

"There are some controversies about this work, and you should probably read about the fine details, Rich. Some researchers have detailed further subdivisions of the anterior cingulate; the functions of the anterior cingulate associated with athletic performance may be further subdivided into a *rostral* (toward the nose) aspect and a *caudal* (toward the tail) aspect. Rostral anterior cingulate functions include most of those that I've been talking about, such as giving feedback to a person when his plans are going astray and need changes. The caudal anterior cingulate may actually be involved in facilitating the effortless present. This region has many connections to the motor cortex and even to the spinal cord, so its activation may serve as a gatekeeper to keep a finely tuned athlete humming without involvement of the rostral anterior cingulate."

Roland paused, and seemed to be thinking what he would say next. Then he looked at me and smiled slightly, as though he were being distracted by something internal. He closed his eyes to rest.

As Roland spoke, it became increasingly clear to me that the unconscious brain response to danger, conflict, and incorrect moves has obvious survival value. We stop ourselves from doing dangerous things, even before we know why we're stopping ourselves. This is why the *feeling of no* over a golf shot is often correct, or why a swing that feels bad usually is. There is something that we are not consciously seeing or feeling that our anterior cingulate is trying to push into our awareness. This activation can be very helpful when standing over a putt: The *feeling of no* is usually an alert to be aware that a slope or grain is not being fully considered. Jack Nicklaus stood over the ball for such a long time sometimes because he continued to see new information about a putt, and he honored this input to the point that he would not putt until he was certain he no longer needed to process anything new. The extent to which a golfer should honor this *feeling of no* probably varies considerably, depending upon the importance of the putt: If it's a putt to determine whether you qualify for the PGA Tour, you should probably wait as long as you need to, although waiting too long will begin to activate other concerns, such as whether you'll be penalized for undue delay. However, if you're playing socially, social concerns will (or should!) make you aware of the social dangers of waiting too long, so it's best to close the gates to new information pretty quickly.

While anterior cingulate activation can alert us to danger, it can also shift us out of focus. One of the cardinal rules of golf instruction is not to have a swing thought that includes the word *no*. This is not just superstition, but rather a deliberate effort not to activate the sputtering negativity of the anterior cingulate. One of the main purposes of engraining the takeaway or the feeling of the club at the top of the swing is so those feelings will be so familiar that no inappropriate *feeling of no* will interrupt the fluidity of the swing.

Demonstrations of the disruptive nature of mounting anterior cingulate activity can be found in many athletic moves that are impaired by hesitation. A golfer who gets caught considering various possibilities for a shot and doesn't commit to one of them, or who begins to think about how a shot will be perceived by others, will almost always be disappointed in the result. The same is true for any athlete who hesitates in producing an action. One of the most striking examples is the basketball player who suddenly finds himself with a wide-open shot, hesitates, and, then, despite the absence of a defender, throws up a herky-jerky jumper that misses. The anterior cingulate activity is producing consideration of alternatives or self-monitoring at a time when the focus should be on releasing the appropriate motor program.

Michael Jordan described how his poor performance led him to doubt himself, and then become stuck in the self-monitoring mode during one of the first games of his second return from retirement, in which he missed his first fourteen shots: "You miss a few and it starts working on you mentally. You start trying to find the mechanics and get more technical during the course of the game—and that's the worst way to come out of a shooting slump. You get confused." Jordan also noted that the way he tries to get out of this mode is to have experiences that will renew his confidence and his focus on letting his play feel effortless: "You try to get free throws, you try to get layups," he said. "You try to get simple things to get your rhythm back."

One of the things that has made Michael Jordan such a strong competitive athlete has been his ability to maintain the right level of motivation and focus on the court. He has been able to control his monitoring system at crucial times in a game, and allow his play to spring to life in front of him, clearly surprising himself at times. For many athletes, the process is not nearly as smooth; some would-be athletes have such trouble reducing the self-monitoring activity of the anterior cingulate that they take themselves out of competition at an early age. The inability to control this mechanism leads to anxiety and fear, which can be debilitating. Many children enjoy sports activities when they are younger but, when the activity is infused with the tension associated with games, or coach or parental pressure, the joy of the activity is reduced or eliminated. Many young athletes turn away from sports at a young age because they no longer experience the joy of the activity. A friend of mine talked about how she loved basketball practice in high school and was one of the best players on the team, but she hated the games, and found that she played terribly whenever she was under the spotlight of competition. She would have liked to stay on a practice track that did not include the games. When she was told she would no longer be a member of the starting five, she felt relieved. If she had been able to properly monitor her increase in anxiety during competition, she could probably have continued to enjoy playing. Some of the techniques that sport psychologists use are essentially efforts to reduce the activation of the anterior cingulate in response to perceived fear.

Roland was now sleeping, having tuckered himself out with his sudden frenzy of intellectual and emotional energy. I had several questions for him, and wanted to wait for him to awaken so I could ask them. How can we control the *feeling of no* so that it's active when we need to increase the extent to which we monitor our performance, yet not active when we want to allow our performance to spring to life in front of us? I suspected our self-consciousness could be diminished through imagery that controls expectation. I also wondered how spontaneous generation can be nurtured in developing children by inhibiting inappropriate responses in a way that won't be associated with fear but, rather, with the expectation of success.

~

As I sat in his hospital room, dusk came and I did not know how long Roland would sleep. He had had no visitors while I was there, and I found this curious. I had never inquired about Roland's personal life, but I always assumed that he had a family and a community of close friends who longed to be in his presence as I did. I did not want to leave. I felt I should be there when he awakened, and I knew he had plenty more to tell me. I jotted down some notes about what he had told me earlier, but the darkness of the room made my notes difficult to read. I turned on a light to see them, but this awakened Roland with a start. He sat upright in his bed.

"Where was I?" he asked, acting fully awake, but seeming a bit disoriented.

I decided to tease him a little and challenge his ability to jump into the conversation as easily as he was pretending he could. I had written down some questions for him, so I read two of them verbatim from my notes.

"If fear and self-consciousness activate the anterior cingulate, and diminish the experience of the effortless present, then what is the effect of changing expectations? Is it possible that developing a clear image of a positive outcome will reduce the anterior cingulate and the monitoring systems of the brain, and allow the motor system to freewheel?"

He gave me a vacant stare, then widened his eyes and rolled them around in their sockets for a second as if to stretch his brain. He looked at me again, this time with his usual intensity, plus a twinge of disdain and annoyance.

"— you," he snarled. I wasn't sure if he was kidding. "Let's all bust the balls of the dead man. I know you've been secretly hoping for this day, when I would become weak and you could spear me in my soft spots."

He paused again for a minute, looked up at me to raise his eyebrows devilishly in rapid succession, then paused for another couple of minutes before he enacted the plan that he had been hatching.

"*Furthermore*," he declared with confidence, "recent brain research has investigated the effect of expectations on the brain. The visual system in the brain operates in a way whereby viewing objects in different places in the outside world activates different regions of the brain. The different places are referred to as *receptive fields*; as you stare out that window, the upper-right corner of the window occupies a different receptive field than the lower-left corner of the window. Decades of research in humans and monkeys have clearly demonstrated that the receptive fields in the outside world can be mapped directly onto specific regions of the brain. The appearance of an object (a fly, for example) on the upper-right receptive field would activate a different part of the visual system in the brain than would the appearance of an object on the lower-left receptive field. Our other domains of perception appear to operate in a similar fashion, and receptive fields for hearing, touch and movement have been studied extensively. Work at the National Institute of Mental Health and our lab here suggests that the brain regions involved in perception become active during the *expectation* of perception. For example, if subjects in the brain scanner are instructed to pay attention to a particular part of a computer monitor that occupies a certain receptive field in their vision and, thus, expect to see something there, they will have increased activations in the brain regions responsible for actually seeing things in those receptive fields. This is how our neural circuitry increases the likelihood of our seeing what we're expecting. These findings provide a neural explanation for countless adages suggesting a relationship between believing and seeing, asking and receiving. We are much more likely to see what we are looking for, and not see what we are not looking for."

"Ask and you shall receive," I muttered.

"Shut up," he said with a smirk. "Some studies extend these research findings in an interesting way. If subjects are told to look at an array of dots on a computer monitor, and to expect to see motion in some of the dots, the regions of the brain responsible for directional motion will become active as the subjects anticipate the movement. If the subjects are told that the motion will be in a specific direction, the activation in *all* these regions will be more active. The anticipation of a specific visual stimulus results in the entire visual system becoming more active. Thus, we not only see what we are trained to expect but, if we expect something very specific, the activity of our entire visual system becomes intensified."

The results he was talking about reminded me of the sport psychology techniques of visualization, and seemed to explain why imagery exercises appear to be more effective if the images are as specific and detailed as possible.

"Our motor system works similarly," he continued. "The expectation to move in a particular manner activates the regions of the motor cortex that are responsible for that movement. This finding was initially a surprise. You know Greg McCarthy, right?"

Greg was the director of the Brain Imaging and Analysis Center at Duke, and I knew him well. We had collaborated on a few fMRI studies together.

"Well, he and Amishi Jha did a study in which they expected to find activation in the areas of the prefrontal cortex involved in planning and preparing to make a movement, which they found. However, they also found activation in the motor cortex, which was not expected, and suggested that the motor system works similarly to the visual system, in that the intention to move in a certain way activates the areas of the brain that are responsible for that movement. Some of this research has served to deemphasize the role of the prefrontal cortex; the plans to move are represented in the regions responsible for movement, not just in the prefrontal, executive part of the brain. In fact, it may be that the accumulation of neural activity in very specific regions of the motor system leads to the decision whether or not to make a movement. It had previously been thought that decisions were the domain of the executive centers of the brain, not the motor cortex. So, all of this work is really changing the way we understand brain function. It's a tremendously exciting time. . . ."

His voice trailed off, but I was too inspired by his ideas to hear the sudden sadness in his voice, weighted by the impending collision between his thirst for knowledge and his impending death. As if summoned by a *deus ex machina*, a nurse appeared to give Roland a bath. I excused myself and headed off to take notes in a waiting area where the television was showing Larry King getting intimate with yet another guest.

The research Roland described had obvious importance to the field of sport psychology. Since the brain is more likely to be specifically active in the regions that are responsible for completing an action, it is best to be very specific in our expectations when we plan to make a move. If the athlete can commit to the action, see exactly what he wants to do, and devote all of his energy to completing the act, his brain will be more likely to activate the specific regions responsible for that action. All golfers have had the feeling of certainty over a shot or a putt that they have seen clearly. If a golfer has lingering doubts about a shot, it is probably due to competition among similar, perhaps neighboring, brain regions. His motor cortex is not active in a specific enough fashion, so he may not have enough of a feeling of certainty. The role of the prefrontal cortex and the anterior cingulate here is to signal the motor cortex that certainty is not high enough and, thus, to deactivate the competing programs. The golfer can then choose the one that stands out the most, and devote all of his brain activity to a single act. This constant interplay between the anterior cingulate, prefrontal cortex, and the motor cortex enables the athlete to develop trust in the *feeling of no* as well as to trust that the absence of this feeling is a green light to proceed effortlessly with his current plans.

According to the research that Roland was discussing, if we expect a certain outcome, and practice seeing this outcome, this will be the guiding principle of our brain's development. If we see failure and have abundant fear, this will be the expectation around which our brain connections develop; the anterior cingulate and the prefrontal cortex will be highly active during our athletic performance, making alternative plans, considering various dangers, and opening us to disastrous outcomes. If we learn to shut down this activity, primarily by pumping up the activity of the relevant motor circuits, the moves can flow out of us like mountain streams in spring. The choice between these alternatives is determined not only by how we decide to approach them, but also by whether we've learned to feel good about generating our own actions.

I was playing golf at a par-3 course with my son, who was then five. When we were on the putting green before our round, after each hole, he yelled his score over to me with great enthusiasm, regardless of what it was: "Dad, I got a three!" he said. "Great!" I replied. "Dad, a two this time!" "Wonderful!" Then, he got a five, and my enthusiasm was not as strong. "Dad, I got a five!" This time, I said only "Okay." He was hurt; his five was not as acceptable to me, he noticed. "Okay? Just okay?" he asked. Later, when we were playing on the course, he became upset because he felt that I was giving more attention to one of our playing partners than to him. As I tried to reassure him, I said, "I love you no matter what shots you hit; I love all your shots." His response revealed that he was still affected by my lukewarm response on the putting green: "No, Dad, you didn't like the five I got on the putting green." Of course, he was right; I didn't like it as much. I didn't want to reward a five with the same enthusiasm that I gave a two or three. The fact is that I didn't love every one of his shots and, at five years old, he was extremely sensitive to this, because he was in the middle of learning how to engage with the world that I was helping to shape around him, learning which ideas and actions would be well received and which would not. It is an important and natural process; we couldn't fit into society if we didn't go through it, but we can't ignore that it squelches our creativity. There is a good chance that my son's next putt will contain a degree of "I hope I don't get a five; Dad will be disappointed. I hope I get a two so that he will be excited!" This is how we learn to generate our thoughts and our actions in the service of how they'll be accepted, in the service of their commercial value. My son, like most kids, has his eyes on my expectations of him as he develops. To the extent that he grows to understand his world and how he can be happy and productive in it, this process is beneficial. However, if his eyes become so fixed on my approval or disapproval that he never develops his own vision, his development will be gnarled and thwarted, and he will eventually become lost and angry.

A Duke wrestler came to me every few weeks to deal with the look he saw coming from his coach. During a match, he would become consumed with how the coach perceived him, and frequently looked over at his coach, sometimes in the middle of a hold. The young man hadn't had a father, and received paternal attention from his high school coach only after he'd established himself as an excellent wrestler. Thus, he viewed his worth as dependent upon his performance and, when his performance was in question, his concern for his worth intensified. This internal dynamic produced in his mind ugly images of being pinned and, at times, on the mat he would become unfocused and distracted. While this process was exaggerated in this particular athlete, to some degree it is present in almost all of us. Athletes are often asked by coaches to *dig down deep* when they're in important situations. According to the brain research that Roland had described to me that day, whether they'll find a vein of riches or an empty hole will depend largely upon the neural circuitry they were given, and how those circuits have been affected by how they've been trained to see themselves.

For many college and high-school athletes, how others see them can be distracting. Dealing with the intrusions of the anterior cingulate may feel at times like learning to ride a bucking bronco. Any signal from the outside world that they're not performing well leads to an explosion of self-monitoring, which can severely disrupt their ability to play well. Many parents and coaches have come to me completely frustrated with tremendously gifted young athletes who seem to lose focus or act like they're unmotivated in these circumstances. Even the athletes may describe themselves as losing intensity. Yet, these periods of apparently low motivation are often due to the athlete shutting down in response to being overly stimulated and emotional. Back in the days before antipsychotic medications, patients with schizophrenia who became increasingly psychotic and excited would have periods of catatonia in which their brains were racing, yet they would stand frozen in one position, sometimes for days, until exhausted. Some died. Young athletes who shut down in response to aroused self-monitoring are similarly reducing their internal stimulation by becoming less intense. A spark of self-criticism leads to a brushfire in the anterior cingulate and prefrontal cortex, and the athlete becomes consumed with thoughts about what she should or should not do, and is unable to simply allow her athletic activity to spring out of her.

According to Roland, one of the primary challenges of human development from adolescence to adulthood is learning when to activate and when to disengage this prefrontal system. To the young adult, since this prefrontal monitoring system is the last to develop, it's the most unfamiliar system of brain activation, and the trickiest for him or her to understand. The athlete has to learn how to move from seeing herself and her performance from the perspective of others (outside-in), to experiencing her performance through the feeling of focus on the action itself (inside-out). Children spend a good deal of time being told what not to do until the lessons from parents, caretakers and teachers are internalized; moving from outside-in to inside-out is the progression from dependent child to independent adult, and those who progress through this development fully are more content and happy in their adult lives. Athletics, especially competitive events, require the participants to move regularly between these perspectives; this may be the aspect of sport that most facilitates growth in young people. Self-efficacy and confidence are a part of this development as well; the young person who can stay within her own perspective and learn that success can be generated from it, will begin to believe in her abilities without the feedback of others. This is the developmental process that facilitates the creativity of greatness.

~

I HAVE TWO GOLFING FRIENDS who have never met. One is a psychotherapist; the other is the president of an advertising company.

Each of them has a tendency to describe some of his shots as *commercial*. The psychotherapist describes as commercial his mediocre shots, while the advertising president uses the word for his best shots. The emphasis that each of them places on the opinions of others about his performance and ideas differs similarly. The advertising president loves to sell people on things, whether it is his shot, his life, or why you should get over a disappointment. He is a tremendously enjoyable partner on the golf course; he is constantly upbeat and tries to establish a positive context in which to view him, his family, and even your own experiences while you are with him. The psychotherapist, on the other hand, seems to view with disdain the notion of ideas as commodities that require selling, as if this puts a blight on the creative process.

Everyone is different in their attitudes toward the relation of creativity and commerce. There is a natural progression from the creation of an idea to its expression and acceptance by the outside world. On the golf course, I have often been very afraid of what my so-called consumers will think of my shots, and of me. This is particularly common on the first tee, when I want my playing partners or bystanders to see my best shot. At my home course, I sometimes hit a driver, even though a three-wood is really the best play for me; I have this vague, barely perceptible notion in the back of my mind that others will think I can't hit my driver. Many of my best ideas have been strangled as saplings—given a few moments to grow, then dug up and discarded or sprayed with toxins. The process of commercializing my ideas can creep too far back into the process of their development. While there is nothing wrong with the commercialization of ideas, it is better placed at the end of the creative process.

This ideal process from creation to commercialization swims upstream against how the world works these days. We have developed into a society of observers where commentators not only affect how we view the world, but also how we think of ourselves. Bobby

Jones had feared that the development of technology allowing golfers to view their own swings would ruin golf, as people would be unable to swing naturally if they knew how they looked from an observer's perspective. For some golfers, he may have been right: Young golfers and other athletes have told me that they think about themselves the way a broadcaster would describe them. The external, outside-in perspective is often strong, and the *broadcaster within* can intensify their self-monitoring when their performance is most crucial, which is usually the time they need it least. This may explain why the television audience prefers the blunt Johnny Miller to any other golf broadcaster, yet PGA Tour players become enraged with him: He gets into their head at times they need to be uncritical, when they need to allow themselves to create without regard to what others think. In many ways, this dynamic between player and broadcaster reflects the ways in which the media, as an expression of community values, determine what's valued, and thus how we value ourselves. Yet those athletes who have enough confidence to stick with the creativity of the moment, regardless of the swirl of analysis and the sweep of criticism around them, will be the money players.

Nothing is more valuable than the present before us. I once discussed the importance of the present with a religion professor at Duke, who quoted Jesus's statement that those complaining of Caesar's taxes were misdirected. The professor said that "give to Caesar what is Caesar's and to God what is God's," refers to the sacredness of the current moment. Money is just a promise of something external in the future; the current moment is here, in front of you, and it is *yours*. No one can buy it or take it away from you. No matter how impoverished or how wealthy you are, you still have the moment that is in front of you, and the richness of this moment exceeds all things financial. Although this biblical passage has been interpreted in a lot of different ways, one interpretation is that we should not be so distracted by the external aspects of life, the packaging holding promises for the future. We should honor our moment-to-moment attention, what is before us, and its connection to divine creation. Become absorbed in this above all else.

When viewed from this secular perspective, the advice of Jesus and Buddha rest on common ground. Prayer and meditation both facilitate focus on the present. They also pay homage to a greatness beyond ourselves, allowing this present to unfold in meaningful ways. If we are not blessed with all of our neurons lined up so that we experience life this way, what can we do? How can we shut down the chattering of the anterior cingulate in those times we don't need it? By giving to God what is God's: the moment of creativity in creation before us.

~

THE AFTERNOON HAD TURNED to evening, and it was now late. The bustle of the corridors had waned, and the absence of motion at the Cancer Center seemed sad. So did Roland. He was so enthusiastic about life, some part of his advanced brain surely wanted to deny that it was coming to an end. I could tell he wanted to talk on into the night, but when I came back into his room, he had again grown tired. I wanted to hear what he had to say to me; he had started out talking about how my book needed to take people farther along, and while he had told me how brain development in children enables the experience of the effortless present, he hadn't said as much about what adults can do toward this end. Somewhat reluctantly, I said goodnight to him, fearing that I would not see him again.

"It could happen any day, you know," he said as I shook his hand with both of mine.

"I'll be back tomorrow," I replied softly.

The next morning, as I drove to the hospital, I had an elaborate fantasy that, when I walked into his room, I saw that all of his things had been removed, and I concluded that he had died, even though he had just changed rooms. Then, in the fantasy, I went distraught back to my office and went about my business, only to find out several weeks later that Roland had not died until a week before. My mind was telling me to be careful of negative expectations.

Roland was indeed alive, awake, and reading the newspaper when I arrived, but he looked a little more tired and pale than he had been the day before. His body was weakening, but the fire was still in his eyes.

"Good morning to be alive!" he exclaimed as I walked in the door.

"It's beautiful out there today," I remarked.

"Is it?" he said with genuine enthusiasm, as if the weather were the most fascinating subject he had ever considered. "I'll bet you'd love to be out there playing golf today, wouldn't you?"

I nodded.

"More than being cooped up here talking about the brain?" he asked.

"I like doing both . . . a lot," I replied emphatically.

"Yes, yes, I know what you mean. I feel like a dog playing with several tennis balls today. I want to jam as many of them in my mouth as possible. I can get about two in there, but every time I go for the third, one of the other ones falls out. Just want to take it all in, take in even more than there is!"

He folded his newspaper and sat up in his bed, alert, emanating energy.

"I thought a lot last night about what I want to tell you," he said with excitement. "It's all about the *effortless present*—I love that term! Did you make it up?"

I reminded Roland that it was a term he used years ago in his discussions with me. I had seen academicians claim to have developed terms or ideas that someone else had communicated to them first, but I had never seen it happen in the opposite direction before; I wondered whether he was naturally modest or being touched by dementia.

"Oh, no wonder I love it so much!" he exclaimed, laughing at himself. "But it's not only about how full attention to the moment before us lets us act effortlessly, but about how *giving* becomes effortless when we're engaged with the moment of what we're doing. We give to the moment; it gives back. We connect with the people before us; they return the gift, the present. It isn't a favor for which we owe each other; it's a present—spontaneous and effortless!"

I had used the term so many times, but I'd never thought of it in this exact light.

"Anyway," he said, keeping the excitement in his voice, "this whole subject is about learning to let go of control when you don't need it anymore. The outside world can seem so benevolent when you do that. Mental practice like meditation, prayer, visualization— all that stuff—just allows us to reap the rewards of every moment. Everything we need is right there in front of us!" He laughed loudly and then smiled at me.

I had done a little research on brain function and meditation, and was excited that he was interested in talking about this, especially since most of the discussions I've had with people about meditation seem to get wacky real fast. Although Roland seemed about to launch into a full manic episode, I expected his approach to be tempered by his scientific background. "I remember you telling me a few years ago that meditation serves to shut down the self-monitoring systems of the prefrontal cortex and the anterior cingulate," I said, jumping into the academic side of the subject abruptly. "When I've meditated, afterward I sometimes feel like I can just act without hesitating and sputtering as much, like I don't need to dwell over various alternatives."

"That's right!" he said, not letting my academic tone deter his enthusiasm. "There have been a few studies showing that when subjects are asked to listen to something they can barely hear or to watch for something they can barely see, they try to clear their minds of any conscious content so they won't miss what's coming. They wait watchfully, not doing, not acting. In many ways this momentary mental state reflects the present-state focus of meditation."

I was glad that he was generalizing the thought processes involved in meditation, rather than presuming that there were mysterious forces involved in its practice. "It's also the gap of time in which a golfer waits for his shot to be released," I added, wanting to make golf a part of the discussion on this crisp and beautiful blue-skied morning.

"Yes," he agreed, nodding with his full body, which made his bed shake slightly. "The functional imaging studies have shown that this period of watchful waiting is accompanied by a reduction in activity within the prefrontal cortex and anterior cingulate. A lot of spiritual disciplines may enhance our ability to reduce the self-monitoring systems in the brain and, thus, allow any activity, especially athletic activity, to spring to life in the effortless present. But before we talk about that further, you have to realize that the more someone practices something, anything, the more the brain changes to let that activity be automatic and engrained.

"The dorsal prefrontal cortex has great influence on the motor system through its specific connections to the premotor cortical areas. When people need to pay attention to their actions, or hold them in mind before they carry out the act, the dorsal prefrontal cortex is engaged and active. If the dorsal prefrontal cortex could talk, it would say many things, but one of its favorite phrases would be 'this is what I am going to do.' It is the seat of intention. When people have learned sequences of activity so fully that they become automatic, the intensity of their intention decreases, and the activity of the dorsal prefrontal cortex and anterior cingulate cortex diminishes."

"Like a golfer engraining a new swing?" I asked, almost harping on the golf theme that was tugging at my sleeve.

"Sure," he said, "any new activity, a quarterback learning a new method of dropping back into the pocket, a pitcher working on a new delivery; it doesn't matter. When people learn the rhythm of a sequence of acts that comprise an athletic move, there are increases in the dorsal premotor cortex and medial frontal cortex (also referred to as the *supplementary motor area* or SMA). Only when a person can perform those acts with precise timing, as required by any complex athletic activity like a golf swing, are these regions active; if the person is constantly responding to the external world in making the moves, or if the complex sequence is experienced as a set of individual acts—like a golfer thinking of his swing in terms of the different positions he needs to attain—the SMA is less active and the prefrontal regions are more active. The more engrained an athletic move is, the more the subcortical parts of the brain such as the cerebellum and the basal ganglia will also get in on the act. That means a highly practiced and repeatable sequence of behaviors becomes the domain of the most primitive and basic structures in the brain. You know the waggle that a lot of golfers use? That may be an attempt to engage these more primitive regions of the brain, to allow the frontal regions to shut down and let the 'unconscious' parts take over.

"If you go back to some of the finger-movement studies, there's a lot in there about how to reduce intentions. Richard Passingham and his group in London have done a series of studies on this subject. In one, they asked subjects to tap their fingers in a certain simple sequence that was either rhythmic or randomly timed. The rhythmic sequences became automatic and flowing, and the subjects began to base their movements on an internal representation of the timing of the sequence. The timing of each finger movement became quicker as the experiment progressed. The randomly timed sequences never became quicker, as they were always a response to the outside world. The brain imaging results from this study indicated that the prefrontal cortex became less active as the finger sequence became automatic. Several other studies have found the same thing, that prefrontal regions become less involved in a task as it becomes learned and engrained. As the subjects engrain the task, the halting sensations of the anterior cingulate are also minimized, and the person can initiate the movement without hesitation, without analysis, without what is experienced as thought. As the activity of the prefrontal, analytical regions diminishes, other regions become more active. The motor regions, which are responsible for the actions, become more active, as do the premotor regions and the supplementary motor area, which are involved in the immediate preparation to take action. As subjects learn to engrain the sequence of finger movements and rely on an internal rhythm to act, the energy devoted to the very specific act of preparing each movement heightens, and this energy is centered on the regions that generate the movement, not the ones that monitor them to see whether or not they're acceptable.

"These studies also suggest that if a task becomes fully learned and engrained into memory, the cerebellum will grow more active. It may be that the cerebellum becomes more active when a person has to work less at analyzing when or how to make a movement. Most studies suggest that the cerebellum is more involved in carrying out an action than it is in making decisions about when or how to act; the role of the cerebellum may be particularly strong in any sequence of actions that has a timed, rhythmic component to it."

The strategy of minimizing effort in the preshot routine reflects this process he described. I remember a professional golfer I worked with saying, "I've got to get the 'try' out of there." He was using his routine to shift his brain activation from the frontal cortex and cingulate to the basal ganglia and cerebellum.

Roland now began to shift the topic. "There is a lot of overlap between the results of these studies on the development of automaticity in complex motor sequences and the results of studies on meditation. First of all, like engraining a complex action, meditation appears to facilitate the experience of action as smooth, automatic, and effortless. Second, the effect of meditation on brain function is similar to the effect of overlearning an action. Each of these activities allows a person to experience motor behavior as a process of having intentions resolved as if of their own accord."

Although Roland's impromptu seminars were always captivating, he had talked to me about some of this before, and I sensed that he was again making sure that I had the background for what he really wanted to say.

He described to me some things that I already knew about meditation, such as that the varieties of meditation are as diverse as the many cultures from which they sprung. Some forms of meditation practice aim to narrow attention to specific contents of the mind or specific perceptual experiences. Other forms aim to broaden attention, and serve to open the mind to supposedly higher states of awareness. These different forms of meditation have been found to have different effects on brain function, with meditation techniques that broaden attention, and require practitioners to reduce willful, effortful action, seeming to deactivate the frontal regions, particularly the dorsolateral prefrontal cortex and the anterior cingulate. Meditation serves to give the brain experience in shutting down its mechanisms for consciously initiating action. Since repeated activity probably generates new growth between neurons, the repeated experience of deliberately reducing the activation of these regions through meditation may generate neural connections that will be a part of a system that aids the initiation of action without interference from the neurons involved in self-monitoring. Through meditation, the brain may actually grow in such a way to facilitate the effortless present.

As discussed earlier, during meditation practice, the meditator allows the images of intention that arise to be released. This meditative state allows practitioners to reduce their anxiety about the outcome of any action; neural processes can then flow smoothly from expectation to intention to the resolution of intention. A golfer in a similar state of mind is able to free himself from the desire for the outcome so he can allow the image of the outcome to be resolved in the external world. However, the golfer-meditator must go through the steps of reminding himself to allow that process to unfold without interference. The relationship between emotion and memory is crucial here, since an overcharged emotional system will reduce an individual's ability to recall memories that may seem out of context. Many athletes become so overwhelmed by the moment that they forget to maintain a focus on releasing intentions. A Duke tennis player who worked diligently on being able to access an open, focused, waiting state of mind described to me after a tournament that he had become consumed with an opportunity to break his opponent's serve, which would send him on to the finals. He became completely unable to focus properly, and lost his patient mindset on the court. The result was a halting, impulsive, overly aggressive style of play, which would have led to defeat if he hadn't looked down at the butt end of his racket, where he had penned a reminder to return to a present-state focus.

In golf, meditation facilitates the feeling of being a mere vehicle for the shot, reducing the self-monitoring that can interfere with our focus on the current moment. While some people are born with the neural circuitry that makes the experience of the effortless present come naturally, and others develop it in childhood and adolescence, the functional imaging results that Roland described to me show how repeated mental exercises, like meditation, can tailor the brain to facilitate this type of experience. The repeated diminishing of the anterior cingulate with its self-monitoring and *feeling of no*, the reduction of the planning and analytic functions of the prefrontal cortex, and the increased expectation for a particular perception to be present in the environment, all come together to heighten and enliven the specific neural circuitry needed in the motor cortex and the cerebellum to bring an intended action to fruition. In this way, a particular shot or putt can seem to be generated on its own.

This process is not limited to golf. For instance, Olympic archers often train themselves to focus intensely on their target while they wait for the proper times to release their arrows. The result of this practice is reduced left hemisphere activation and decreased heart rate just prior to release of the arrow.

If neuroscience taught us only this much about how reducing the activation of the prefrontal cortex and the anterior cingulate affects athletic performance, our understanding of sport psychology would certainly be enhanced. Yet, I felt there was a more general and relevant effect that could be gleaned from this work, and that Roland intended to lead me there.

"So, what is there in this that you feel I should communicate to everyone in this book, you know, to get beyond the foothills?" I asked.

"It's not just golf and athletic performance," he replied, echoing my wife's declaration of years ago. "The universality of these effects is far more impressive. After all, meditation is generally pursued as a spiritual discipline, not to enhance performance. There is some recent evidence that meditation, prayer, and other mental disciplines change the brain in such a way that the experience of *where* we are is reduced, and our ability to understand the experience of other people is dramatically increased."

For the first time in our discussion, I could see a mountain peak jutting out ahead. Roland had become subdued and serious, and each of his sentences was deliberate. I took notes.

"Meditation helps reduce an exaggerated concern for the outcome of our actions by literally reducing the intensity with which we experience ourselves as being where we are. It is likely that this experience enables us to engage with the outside world more fully. Various forms of meditation have been found to reduce activation in the parietal cortex, which is responsible for processing spatial information and establishing a person's sense of orientation. This reduction in activation may be associated with the spiritual experience of the loss of boundary between the self and the greater outside world. As a person's sense of orientation diminishes, the person feels less localized to his current place. One of the natural outcomes of feeling less oriented, less physically localized, is to feel more oriented outside oneself. This shift in orientation may easily result in the meditator feeling more connected to the rest of the universe, known and unknown, and all of the representations of it that the meditator has in mind.

"In one study, brain-imaging data were collected while subjects reported feelings of oneness with the outside world. These feelings were associated with reduced activity in the parietal areas and superior temporal lobule, which are active during the localization and identification of objects in the external world. This shift in brain activity may represent how religious experience is created or perceived.

"Some people may view such research findings as an indication that mystical experience is not real, but just a figment of a brain process. However, this is like saying that what we see is not real, but just a figment of our eye or visual system, since this is the mechanism by which we perceive it. As that religion professor from UNC had said to me years ago, the brain would certainly be a likely candidate to serve as the window through which the glory of God's light shines upon us. This mechanism is in the brain to be utilized; why in the world would we choose on theoretical grounds not to utilize it?"

The ability of the brain to reduce its self-absorption so we can experience empathy for other people was fascinating to me, and I felt like I had just walked out onto a precipice that revealed a new world.

I remembered a bizarre experience I had had. A few weeks after September 11, 2001, my wife and I took our children to Busch Gardens in Virginia. My son wanted repeatedly to go on rides that gave us an intense experience of falling. One ride was a huge boat that rocked backwards to front so severely that at the apex, riders were suspended high in the air facing the ground with nothing between them. I usually like these rides, but this time, it was torture. Every time we were suspended in the air and began to plummet toward the earth, I thought of the people who had been in the World Trade Center, and how it must have felt for them to be falling in terror. It was like an overdose of empathy that I could not ignore. I was struck then by how the images we have of others affect our own personal experience. And now, Roland was going to tell me how and why the brain works this way.

"Some recent fMRI studies have demonstrated that when someone watches another person performing an action, it is not just the visual system that's active; also active are the regions responsible for *performing* that action. Everyone has heard of the study in which piano players listening to music activated the regions of their brains that move their fingers when they play the piano, even though, in the scanner, their fingers were perfectly still. But, there are a lot of other similar findings. Studies of facial perception show that when we look at someone expressing an emotion, the areas that are active are very similar to those active when we *experience* that emotion. If I look at your face, and you look disgusted, the areas in my brain that experience disgust will become active! What all this research is telling us is that we understand others in part by feeling what it would be like to be them. We don't have to try to be sympathetic to other people; it is how we understand others' actions, feelings, and intentions. It is how we experience empathy. Through meditation, the brain appears to reduce its focus on self-experience, and opens a window for this type of empathic experience. No wonder all great religions view the experience of empathy as the crowning achievement of discipline and faith: The more we engage in religious practices such as meditation and prayer, the more we reduce our ongoing attention to the self, and the more we enhance our neural systems that allow understanding and empathy.

"We appear to be wired with the potential to feel what we see. We can understand how others feel and why they do what they do, because when we watch them our own neural patterns of feeling and doing are activated."

This explanation of the neural circuitry of observation and empathy dovetailed nicely with the reports of some athletes who described confusion between imagery perspectives. They said that when they tried to take a third-person perspective—seeing one's self from a distance—it often switched into first-person imagery—feeling one's movements.

The brain may be delicately designed to enhance learning by watching, which also engenders feelings of empathy in some people. Roland explained that the causes of this difference are not really understood: "As we know from social interactions, some people are very good at empathizing with, and understanding, other people, while others seem completely incapable of it. It's unclear whether this capacity is genetically hardwired or whether it stems from social interaction. Most likely, it's both. We are probably born with the neural capacity to feel what others are feeling just by observing them, yet this is only fully realized if it's nurtured from the early stages of life. Children will do a thousand cruel things during their childhood, at least mine did. I remember, when they were small, always being poised between fostering discipline through fear, like saying, 'Do that again and I will smack you,' and doing what seemed harder sometimes in trying to develop their empathy by saying, 'How would you feel if someone did that to you?' I think that people often misunderstand empathy. They sometimes mistake it for softness of heart. I always feel the opposite. Having a good idea of how someone feels is knowledge and power. Knowing the feelings and intentions of others enables us to make the choice to support them or protect ourselves from them if need be.

"When we engage in activities that reduce our self-concern, the brain regions involved in orientation are reduced. This allows an experience of connection to the world we see outside of us, and to the plight of the people who live in that world. This state of mind, which can be achieved under various circumstances, facilitates a focus on the richness of the stimuli before us and the actions in which we're engaged. It facilitates our ability to understand other people and have our intentions resolved."

With that statement, Roland closed his eyes and fell asleep. As I waited for him to awaken, I, too, fell asleep, and I had a disturbing dream that I was in a disco in Beirut, dancing with Osama bin Laden.

~

THE PROCESS of having our intentions resolved sometimes seems far beyond our control. We ask and receive, yet how we come to receive seems arbitrary and inexplicable. It was not at all clear to me how the brain could be involved in allowing us access to a more universal state of being, if indeed there is one. I wanted to hear more from Roland, but he had finished his latest treatment, and had gone home.

He called me the next week and asked me to come over to his house. It would be our last conversation. He looked frail and drawn, and seemed to have lost a lot of weight in only a few days. As though his time and energy would soon be gone, he wasted no time getting to the points he wanted to make to me: "Some people talk about heaven," he said, "or living in states of bliss that last an eternity, but I don't really believe them. I mean, I don't know if they're deluded or just lying. The real world is littered with tripwires and mines, and any direction will eventually need adjustment. When we are cruising on automatic pilot, sometimes we're dead wrong. We have to be snapped out of our reverie, be forced to pay attention to the mismatch of our plans and what we should be doing.

"Thank God for the ventromedial prefrontal cortex, which helps us recognize these breaches in expectation! It allows us to be flexible and adapt to the shifting contexts and perspectives inherent in a changing world. On the other hand, when we're correct in the direction of our intentions, it is sometimes more efficient for us to proceed uninterruptedly, even to remain unaware of how our intentions are resolved, so that we'll refrain from looking at ourselves and disturbing the process of resolution. However, the decision to trust ourselves or to be jolted from our erroneous reverie is very —ing complex."

He slammed his fist into his other open hand when he said this, as if he were not only frustrated with the complexity of the brain processes, but also with the fact that he knew he'd never have the chance to understand them fully.

"When we have explicit knowledge of something, we are correct about it 100 percent of the time. When we have no knowledge, we are guessing. In between these, we sometimes have implicit knowledge of something—that is, we know without knowing that we know, and we have the feeling that we know. Other times, we think we know, but we're just guessing. The fact that we can confuse implicit knowledge with guessing has a dramatic impact on our willingness to use implicit knowledge. Many people shut down their ability to access implicit knowledge because they'd rather depend on what is rationally knowable than look to an undependable source of information. They're afraid! The uncertainty of implicit knowledge makes some people feel insecure, so they try to ignore it. But other people, the real tough angels of the world, do the opposite: Despite the heart-searing consequences, they open themselves up *even more* to this unknown process in the world. All of those mental exercises we've talked about, whether meditation or prayer or imagery or playing golf, they activate the same brain mechanisms as accessing and acting upon implicit knowledge!

"There have been a lot of studies of this in the past few years. They use computerized tests such as words of colors being presented just before patches in different colored ink. Subjects are shown the word *red* or *green*, and then a color patch that is either red or green. Sometimes the words and the ink are congruent, like the word *green* followed by a color patch in green ink, and sometimes they are incongruent, as when the same word *green* is followed by a color patch in red ink. The subjects are told to indicate as quickly as possible the color of the patch. Some studies have shown that when the word before the color patch is congruent with the patch, reaction time and accuracy get better, even when the word is shown so quickly that the subjects say they are unaware of what the word is. You get it? People can get smarter without having any idea of how or why they are more effective!

"In one of the recent studies, the methods were a little different, and the results suggested that people act very differently if the unconscious information is a warning sign or an indication to proceed. For one part of the study, the words and colors were incongruent 75 percent of the time, and were presented slowly enough to be processed consciously. The result was that subjects used this information to improve. They learned that the word *green* was associated with the red patch, and increased their accuracy and reaction time for the *incongruent* words. However, in another part of the study, when the information was presented too quickly for explicit processing, yet was processed implicitly—unconsciously—the subjects continued to be tricked by the incongruence between the word and the color, and were slower for the incongruent words only! You see, in the other studies, the congruent associations could be learned implicitly, and help people react quickly, but in this one, people were never able to stop the danger of the incongruence between the words and the colors from slowing their reactions unless they got this information explicitly.

"This shows that conscious and unconscious perception of the same stimulus information can lead to very different behaviors. Are you understanding this? Unconsciously perceived information leads to automatic reactions that cannot be controlled by a perceiver. Conscious perception allows people to use the perceived information to guide their actions so that they can react to stimuli in a more flexible manner. If we only unconsciously perceive the tripwires and landmines, we will get scared for what seems to be no reason; sometimes we'll freeze, and sometimes we'll go ahead and blow ourselves to pieces. Yet, if there are aspects of the environment that help us, and we're not conscious of them, we'll still be able to use them to our advantage. The process of functioning without conscious awareness of the functions that are operating is of course more efficient than being aware of every little intention, every little move we make. So, *not* becoming aware of how we resolve some of our intentions, as long as the processes continue to be effective, is much better than making these processes conscious. Sometimes, it's *better* to be unconscious! We just have to figure out when these times are!

"The state of mind reflected by this process, enhanced by meditation and reported by athletes in the zone and by mystics for millennia, is elemental to our existence. We all have it, but we rarely talk about it. We intend, and our intentions are resolved without conscious effort. A rudimentary form of this skill, to be able to resolve our intentions, has probably been around for a long time—at least three and a half billion years, back to when life began on this planet. We've had all this time to become expert at figuring out what we want by developing a clear internal picture of it, then moving toward that picture in the outside world. This is the primary function in our lives, and it has been so since we were microscopic one-celled organisms flailing around in the primordial soup trying to get the right acid-base balance in our cells. We've developed a superbly adequate body and a brain that enables us to become aware of intentions that are doomed to fail. Any evolutionary biologist will declare that the primary purpose of our evolution, our development into humans, was to facilitate our ability to get what we want in our environment. Look out the window: It is just teeming with life engaged in movement, life nurturing life. Mother to child, child to mother. Effortless and present. Wouldn't it make sense, then, after all this time—with three and a half billion years of development behind us—that we would have found a way to move toward the resolution of our intentions without being fully aware of how they were being resolved? This is the core evolutionary advantage of visualization, intuition, and even mysticism. We are able to have what we want, to be who we want, to live the way we desire, as long as we fully expect the resolution of our intentions to unfold.

"Rich, many reasonable people will recoil and retreat when they hear this. They'll say that it's too bold or too extravagant. Yet, what if it were true that we could manifest whatever we visualized but we never really tried? What if someone had a special gift for this process and he never allowed it to flourish? What if he just stayed, holding on to what he hoped and insisted was right, and he never opened himself up to other possibilities? Is that the perspective of an objective, rational person, or of someone who is just too afraid to let go of an opinion that is keeping him afloat in a sea of uncertainty?"

Roland lay back in his bed and took a deep breath. A healthy pink color had returned to his face, but he looked worn out. As he lay there, he stared at me intently; I didn't know if he was expecting me to answer his questions, or if he was quietly peering into eternity. The air between us was still but not heavy, and time passed by silently but not unpleasantly. Eventually, I got up to leave and hugged him; he patted me firmly on the back. As I drove away, the sweet sting of his hand landing on my back lingered.

A week later, Roland's secretary called me to tell me that he had died. I had never felt more alone or more challenged. He had handed to me a staff I feared I could not carry.

CHAPTER NINE

The Enhancement
of Intimacy

ROLAND'S DEATH AFFECTED every aspect of my life. I had trouble playing golf for quite a while. I still loved the game, and spent a lot of time on the course working with golfers, trying to help them work in the effortless present, to enhance their careers or their enjoyment. Yet I ignored my own game. I frequently heard Roland's words in my mind, and felt that I needed to somehow move beyond golf, to understand how the development of the effortless present can help everyone resolve their intentions. While golf had gotten me here, I began to feel that I should stay away from playing at anything; golf would be a reward for hunkering down and delivering Roland's message. Golf had been my discipline, and I hoped that my moving away from it was only temporary.

When I talked to people about Roland over the years, everyone commented on how brilliant he was, and how driven he was; no one mentioned his personal life. It seemed natural at the time to focus solely on his intellectual energy. The upshot of these discussions was that we all wanted to possess Roland's genius, to be like him—but, if we'd scratched the surface, we probably would not have wanted his life.

I found several people who had been mentored by Roland or had worked with him at some point in his career. His wife had divorced him years ago, and he no longer had contact with her or their two children. Those who knew Roland well eventually chose not to be close to him. He was like a fire burning hot, attractive and warm from a distance, but moving toward him and trying to touch him had eventually left everyone hurt and wary of him. Roland's energy burned on its own; it did not burn for those around him. I was evidently a fortunate recipient of good timing in my relationship with Roland: I had been enthralled enough to learn from him, self-deprecating enough to feel that he did not want to see me any more than he had to, and then only personally involved with him near the end, when he had something he wanted me to tell everyone.

I felt sad for him. He had ideas about how to improve people's lives, and how the brain made this possible, yet he could not fully enjoy the kinds of human interactions his ideas promoted. He was like one of the indigent pearl divers off the cliffs of Mexico: He pierced the depths where others could not go, returned with gems that he could appreciate, but was too poor to be able to keep them for himself.

I began to see Roland's message in everything. While I'd known that the effortless present could be accessed and applied to performance in golf and other sports, I became more fully aware of the view, expressed in philosophical writings for thousands of years, that these moments offer boundless opportunity. It began to strike me that everything we have learned about visualization, the resolution of intentions, and the effortless present could be applied to every moment of life, every day with everyone around us. I began to see the process of the effortless present even in experiences I had had years ago. And I could feel in my life what Roland could not; I longed to enrich every single moment that I would have with other people.

Sport psychology techniques are used by elite athletes to enhance their ability to perform in the realm of their greatest passion. For most of the rest of us, limiting the application of these principles to sport would enhance our enjoyment of a leisure activity. It seems silly for us to stop there, with the whole rest of our lives awaiting us. If we can infuse the effortless present into each shot, what about each task at work, each act of discipline and education with our children, each conversation with our friends and intimate partners?

The focus of our attention in golf and sport is not usually on the importance of emotional connection with other people, yet the real value we take from our athletic endeavors is in the relationships we form along the way. It's ironic that we turn only to winners for vindication of this view; it's as though we feel that, if you or your team did not emerge on top, any satisfaction you obtained from the people along the way is just a rationalization of empty effort. Nonetheless, many athletes and coaches who have won championships have observed upon reaching a lifelong goal that they are far less enthralled with the prize than with the relationships they formed on the way to it. The moments of their greatest victories feel strangely hollow without those closest to them.

Anson Dorrance, whose women's soccer teams at the University of North Carolina won sixteen of the twenty-one NCAA championships played from 1982 to 2002, said that his first victory was shockingly empty for him; it wasn't until the next summer, when he received letters from some of his graduating players saying that they would miss seeing him in the fall, that he began to feel satisfaction. Jimmy Valvano, coach of North Carolina State's surprising basketball champions in 1983, ran onto the court at the end of the final game, dashing about madly, "looking for someone to hug." While victory seems like the worthwhile final goal, the relationships along the way are the substance of the trip. Part of the challenge is for athletes and coaches to allow themselves to feel this way even if they don't become champions.

Relationships are not only part of the spoils of victory, but are on the minds of athletes at times of greatest pressure and greatest anguish. I once played golf with Bobby Thomson, whose three-run home run in the bottom of the ninth inning was the shot heard around the world that gave the New York Giants the National League pennant over the Brooklyn Dodgers in the 1951 playoff. Upon learning of my work in sport psychology, he told me about his mental state as he waited for his final turn at bat that day. In the previous play, Don Mueller had been hurt sliding, so there was a delay in the game, which gave him plenty of time to think about what he was about to do. In the pregame warm-up, he had looked around and thought to himself about his teammates and was overcome with a connection to them. "That Alvin Dark," he said to himself, "I'm glad he's on my side. Look at that Whitey Lockman, what a player he's been for us." By the time he stepped to the plate, the connection with his teammates lingered, and he urged himself on: "Come on you son of a bitch, get back to fundamentals; wait and watch, wait and watch." He had become thoroughly absorbed in the urgency of the moment—not for himself, but for his team.

Even at the lowest times in an athlete's career, he is likely to gain solace from the connections he feels from others. A Duke football player, following a game in which Duke was losing 28-0 at halftime, then came back to tie the game at 35-35, before losing 42-35, said to me: "We'd lost eighteen games in a row, and we're down 28-0. What else is there to play for other than my teammates?"

The connection with other people we can gain from sport is not limited to relationships with teammates. Engaging with our competitors is also enlivening to any athlete who yearns for the effortless present. The rules and traditions of tournament golf establish a particular opportunity for feeling the connection with competitors. When Tiger Woods checked off one of his lifelong goals in 2000 (if someone twenty-four years old can be considered to have anything that is lifelong) by winning the career grand slam at St. Andrews, the expression on his face was curious; not one to contain his excitement or pride, he seemed muted, almost sad. Was something missing? Was his eight-shot victory hollow? Was he disappointed that his friend and competitor David Duval had not put up a better fight? His words argued no, but his face seemed to belie them. The contrast with his expressiveness three weeks later, when he defended his PGA Championship title in a gripping overtime battle with Bob May, was striking; at that moment of victory, he seemed overjoyed and fully alive. He seemed genuinely emotionally connected to May, and hugged his reluctant competitor at the end of their match. Woods says that he would rather win by fifteen strokes than by one, but I don't believe him. Is he keeping the truth from just us, or would it be so anathema to his step-on-your-throat attitude that he needs to keep it from himself as well? I think he loves confrontational competition, the connection with another master who challenges him to a duel. When he wins by twelve strokes, he is lonely. Countless psychology studies have determined that humans who perfect a task will change the task in order to decrease their success rate and increase their interest. Winning seems like enough from a distance but, up close, it is unfulfilling without other people in the mix. Interactions with teammates and competitors facilitate the effortless present by demanding a certain level of attention and motivation; this engagement not only enhances performance, but also invigorates the athlete's experience.

~

ONE TICKLISH AREA of interpersonal interaction in sport is the distinction between being motivated to excel in order to fulfill the desires of others, and being motivated to fulfill desires upon which the athlete and others have mutually agreed.

Many athletes say that they perform better when they're motivated to play for someone other than themselves. To excel, we need to fight through limitation and pain, and striving for our own benefit occupies the same frequency in our brains as our limitation and pain. The neural networks that connect to what we experience as the self are activated by pain; if we suffer, the self-monitoring system of the prefrontal cortex and rostral anterior cingulate become active, and we become too concerned with protecting ourselves to mount and execute a clear, specific plan of attack. We become defensive and afraid. Yet, when we strive for the benefit of someone else, such as father, spouse, teammate, the Gipper (moms are not usually included in this group unless they're sick), a different series of brain regions are activated, and our drive is orthogonal to our pain and limitation. In this manner, we can drive ourselves to achieve what our self-monitoring system would have difficulty allowing us to do. As any military officer or coach will tell you, the energy born from selfless determination far exceeds that of individual agendas.

However, the relationships that form the foundation of motivation for many athletes are not always healthy; sport has seen increasing numbers of children who participate, or even excel, only to please a demanding parent. The common seed in this pathology is the attempt of parents to get their children to live for them. This is not an agreed-upon agenda. While this works very well when children are small, since they lack the knowledge to form an agenda, it becomes a problem if the child does not develop independent views as she grows into an adult. Unfortunately, we hear of the successes of child prodigies far more often than we hear of the numerous failures; a child who feels worthless because he was berated or ignored by a disappointed parent doesn't make the lead story on *SportsCenter*. The PGA Tour player Scott Simpson once suggested to me that "for every Tiger Woods, there are probably a million kids who compete only to please a demanding parent." I have seen many athletes in my office who found that, when they finally grew up enough to think for themselves, they lost their interest in their sport. Quite often, parents of these children were so involved in the child's success as an extension of the parents' egos, that the parents treated the child just like they've treated themselves: demanding, critical, and always dis-

appointed. This type of external motivation does not enhance performance; it keeps people from being who they are, and so impedes
any opportunity to experience the meaningfulness of the effortless
present.

Quite often, interpersonal relationships can drive an athlete and
hold him back at the same time. An amateur golfer named David,
whom I helped with the mental side of his game, described to me the
importance of his family while he was progressing through a series
of matches to win a major national amateur championship. Images
of his family spurred him on and comforted him at times, and yet
these same images almost kept him from attaining the goals that
were important to him and them.

Many kind and supportive strangers surrounded David during
and after the tournament. All of them seemed genuinely interested
in him, and congratulated him on each of his victories, but they took
the tournament very seriously, and he couldn't help feeling that they
had no idea who he really was. He called his family and close friends
throughout the series of matches, which helped, but there were
a couple of people who seemed a little ambivalent about his success. The most disturbing reaction was the dampened enthusiasm
expressed by his younger brother, Steve. David had always over-
shadowed Steve in high school and college, where he played golf and
Steve was cut from the team. David hadn't seen any shame in that,
but Steve was so devastated that he fell into a depression requiring
medication to pull him out of it. Their father had tried to distribute
his attention to them evenly, but his joy in following David's golf
matches and his pride in David's success was obvious. A friend of
David's once told him that, while he was in college, his father said
to David's father, "You must be proud of David when you go to his
golf tournaments." Evidently David's father paused, lit a cigarette,
then stared his friend's father in the eye and said, "It's better than
—ing."

His father had had a rough life, so David was happy his father could enjoy watching him play, but it was overwhelming to David that he was replacing his mother, as it were. His little brother had felt all of this family intensity growing up. When Steve paid more attention to his rock band and hanging around with his friends than to playing sports, he didn't progress as David had, and couldn't quite play at the college level. This was fine with everyone in the family, but Steve didn't get the attention that David had, and he was troubled by it. As David progressed through to the finals of this tournament, he wanted to share his victories with Steve, but he was afraid of what Steve was feeling: Did it pain him to have to give David attention with all the others yet again? Steve was the person David thought of first when he was successful at something; sometimes David would call him so that he would feel a part of it, so he wouldn't feel that David was moving away from him. Sometimes, he heard genuine joy from Steve when he called; other times, Steve seemed to be faking it, or quickly changed the subject to something he had done recently.

Luckily, David had a couple of people in his life who could understand all this and was able to share it with them, which helped him to feel that he wasn't wreaking havoc on his loved ones by winning a few golf matches. It also helped to think about his father: "When it gets really bad with my worrying about Steve, I think of Dad, and how much it means to him, and all he taught me, and it really helps to refocus myself. I guess I feel that closeness with him, and it feels like I'm on the right track after all."

In the end, healthy, supportive relationships allow a return to a present-state focus. They allow an athlete to be who he is and facilitate the effortless present.

~

THE CONCEPTS OF SPORT PSYCHOLOGY, especially visualization, can be applied to develop and enhance our relationships. College athletes are often astounded by the idea of applying visualization to non-athletic parts of their lives, and seem to feel that they need to ask permission to do so: "You mean, I can apply this stuff to *my life*?" Of course, many of these techniques were developed without golf or sport in mind, so their application to things like interpersonal relationships isn't surprising. Few experiences are as satisfying as being in the effortless present together with another person. Intimate conversations, silent understanding, and sex are all examples of interpersonal interactions that are greatly enhanced by becoming fully present with the other person involved. Theologian Martin Buber described the I-You experience as a form of mysticism in which the opportunity for these interpersonal experiences is ripe. Buber described the source of these experiences as divine. Some of the sport psychology techniques and spiritual disciplines that we've discussed enable an experience of the effortless present not just as a means of enhancing performance, but of enhancing intimacy as well.

Each day, an intimate partner is a new person. If we can see our partners as they are today, not as what we remember of them or what we thought they were, we keep the relationship alive. Our tendency is to deaden things, to pretend that we know them and think we don't need to summon up as much energy toward them. When we feel that some aspect of our lives is going well, or at least well enough, we often give it less attention and move on to other things, as if we're executives managing our resources: "Okay, the marriage is going fine, kids are healthy. Good. I'll turn my attention toward my work." Like the process of habituation, we start not to see what's there, and assume that it doesn't change. This is very efficient for some of our perceptual processes (why keep looking at something that doesn't change?), but it's neither accurate nor effective in our relationships. The irony is that we often feel that we're constantly changing, but that our partners don't change at all. The fact is, we see changes in ourselves much more readily than changes in our partners, because it's more comforting to think that we know that partner, and that they don't do things that surprise us. If we give in to this, our relationships become old, stale, and boring, and we wander toward new ones. But there is no status quo in the effortless present. If we pay attention to each moment with our partners, we notice how different they are each day. When we are fully engaged with them, we see them for who they *really* are, new every day.

A friend of mine, upon learning of visualization at a golf psychology seminar, began using it in his marriage. He often became stressed at work, and when he entered his home, he expected to be greeted by a calm wife and happy children running to greet him. He was usually disappointed when he arrived to find them busy and engaged in activities that couldn't be interrupted and, since the children were small, there was often chaos everywhere. He'd get annoyed and disengaged from the family scene, and behaved in ways that added to the chaos. To try to handle this situation better, as he was driving home, he visualized what it would be like to walk in the house. He saw himself walking into the house with his wife haggard and the children yelling and banging toys; he saw himself adding calm to the situation, and lending a hand instead of immediately expecting his stressed-out needs to be met. He feels that this visualization exercise helps him to focus on the current moment, and allows him to be present with his wife and children in a way that ultimately increases everyone's satisfaction.

This technique can be used whenever people are in situations that seem to raise emotions they don't really want or are inappropriate. A husband who had trouble hearing his wife's anxieties, and who got angry when she expressed any kind of negative emotion, acknowledged that his mind would drift to the conclusion that she was unhappy and that he was to blame. When he learned to keep his focus on the current situation and to listen to what she was saying, he found that he was more angered by the disappointment of his expectations than by her emotions and, when he let her talk without interrupting her or blaming her, she felt much better, became calmer, and their interactions improved for both of them.

Once, when I was interviewing a veteran at a Veterans Affairs Hospital during graduate school, he told me about his time in Vietnam, where he had been captured. He was an athlete in high school, and had read a study of imagery. He wound up using imagery intensely throughout his imprisonment.

When I returned from 'Nam, the Army guys wanted to gather information against the enemy, so they completed a series of interviews with me. I think they wanted to justify some of their planned military actions, but I could not help them. When they asked me whether my time in solitary confinement had been difficult, I could only give an answer that was true. I was told that it would have been far more politically expedient to criticize my captors, but I could not bring myself to do so. For, although they had not fed me over the first few days, when I was starving they flashed pictures of my family up on the walls of my dark prison cell. They showed videos of my children playing in our yard at home. And they pumped in the sounds of their laughter and "we love you Daddy" in English! And although my bed was small, they had seemed to shape it in the exact form of my wife's body, and my sleep was deep and comforted. Toward the end of my imprisonment, when other men would have become hopeless, they spoke to me in the exact voice of my mother. And although they seemed not to understand me when I spoke to them, their words to me were comprised only of her encouragement and patience. At times, they used the exact words that she had said to me when I was sick as a child. So, I am unable to criticize them. For when my life was at its darkest hour, they brought to me all that I needed.

The ability to focus on the other may be one of the most evolutionarily rewarded behaviors in the human arsenal. Few other behaviors are more likely to lead to the propagation of the species. A male student who had many relationships over the course of his college years described it to me like this: "How much does a woman love it when a man is totally zoned in on her and can't take his eyes off her and wants her and needs her so much? It's the energy that leads to most of our lives! He says, 'I need you and want you,' and she likes that and eventually if he holds his fix on her long enough and learns to dance with her just like she wants, she says 'yes' and then a baby comes into the world and the genes that said 'I want you' as they were staring in her eyes and the genes that whispered 'yes you can' live on and on. And then some administrator crawls out from under a rock and says you can't feel that way and some ugly woman who never heard the man want her hears the administrator and she tells everyone that it's not fair and then before you know it, it's illegal to have an erection." Or something like that.

The best example I ever witnessed of resolved intentions in interpersonal relationships was with a friend of mine named Gary McKee, who was not normally a confident man. We had a mutual good friend and, years ago when we were single, the three of us used to get together occasionally to go out drinking and try to meet women in New York City. We were overwhelmingly unsuccessful. One day, we went into a bar, grabbed a beer, and settled ourselves against the wall as usual. Then, completely uncharacteristically, Gary said, "Okay gents, sit back, and let 'em come to us." An hour later, he met the woman he would marry.

~

I FIND THAT WHEN I STOP TRYING so fervently to get things done in relationships and unfurrow my frontal cortex a bit, the relationships begin to operate in ways that alarm me and please me. This is comparable to what people describe as God coming into their lives, with wonderful experiences coming to me and love seeming to flow through me. This process has never been more fully expressed than in my marriage. My usual approach to relationships before I met my wife (with apologies to Michael Stipe) was half done, will travel. That searing commitment to another person was never possible for me. When I met my wife, though, our moments together were filled with a larger feeling of meaning, and even our disagreements had a flow and a purpose. At times, I felt like I was just riding along, enjoying the lights and the action. The state of mind was somewhere between trying to change things and ignoring them; it is the same kind of focus as the release of a pured shot. My attention is fully on her, yet the interaction springs to life on its own, without any efforts to steer its direction.

I remember vividly a time when we were at the beach soon after we were married. I looked at her and I realized that she, too, saw the sun setting into the ocean in the same way I did. The pink-orange hues shone like pinpoints in the corner of her eyes. She saw an entire world just as I did, and though this was obvious, when I really *felt* it, I realized that we are all worlds unto ourselves. As Plotinus, the great mystic of the third century, said, "Each being contains within itself the whole intelligible world. Therefore all is everywhere. Each is there all and all is each." When I shut down enough to allow myself to be together with her, the entire world is available in duplicate, side by side, revolving around each other in a dance choreographed by a gravity beyond our control.

I saw it again the other day for a brief, unexpectedly unhurried moment. Walking through the halls of Duke Hospital, where Roland's words continue to echo as a reminder, I allowed myself to just be, to look, and not try. I could almost feel my rostral anterior cingulate shut down, and a world of experience opened before me. I stopped monitoring what I was doing, and I could feel the absence of planning that the frontal cortex insists upon. I saw people looking out for each other. One woman was crying and being physically supported by a man who appeared to be her lifelong partner. Perhaps she had been diagnosed with breast cancer; perhaps her mother had just died. There was a fundamental sadness and tenderness that wafted through the air from them. I felt a passing desire to ease her pain, to soothe her somehow. Down the hall, a man held the door open for an older woman. If he were impatient for her bulky frame to make its way through, he did not show it. Many kindnesses are enacted for the benefit of the person acting; we may want to enhance our position in society or our view of ourselves by being seen as kind and good. The search for legitimate kindness and love can be a shell game; we've become so adept at disguising our selfish interests as benevolence. Yet some kindnesses go beyond this; they are for their own purpose, for the legitimate benefit of the other. At these times, I see the movements of angels in mere men and women. How could we be considered animals when so much of our society is devoted to caring for one another, for looking out for each other?

It hit me on this day that everyone is invited. Your skin can be white or yellow, black or brown, wrinkled or surgically stretched. Your past can be rich with devotion or littered with crimes and betrayals. You are invited. You may have lied to your preacher. You may have cursed your mother as she lay dying. You may have cut yourself with razor blades to distract yourself from your sadness. You may have denied your best friends, and lusted after their wives and children. The invitation still stands; in fact, you cannot be disinvited. You may have won the lottery and pissed it away on cocaine. You may have prayed every day for decades. You may be someone who complains about scratches on your Mercedes-Benz. You are still invited. Everyone is invited to the connection with the rest of us. No one can be banned from the common ground of human love. Ask someone who has raised a deformed child if they would wish for something different. How is it possible that we were built to love like this? Each person has been designed as a separate delivery system of love.

I have been mugged on the streets of New York City: punched in the face, had my glasses shattered into my eyes by the fist of an adolescent boy who cursed the gall I'd shown by looking at him. I have spoken with women whose husbands beat them and chained their hearts to keep them away from the wealth of emotional riches they could not provide. I have seen lost, angry souls blunt the growth of young college athletes, chosen by the rest of us to be terminal gladiators, their dreams half eaten by ravenous mentors. And I still say that we're getting better. The youth of today have been a shaky step from anarchy since civilization began. We now have so many opportunities to be with each other in a way that promotes our interconnection. Slaves died building the Egyptian pyramids. Only a century and a half ago, slaves helped to build mansions and pick the cotton that clothed the country. We now understand universally that this is wrong. Yes, I know that globalization and technology are dangerous bedfellows, and the hateful and greedy can cut through civilization like a thresher through fresh hay. This does not refute our progress, but merely emphasizes its necessity. I believe that we as a species are learning more and more as we go, learning about how to love each other better. This is not the kind of love that is contingent upon the shape of someone's body or another aspect of their gene pool. We are learning how to restrain ourselves from primitive urges that we will never shed. Learning to allow each other to be as we are. Our challenge in the years ahead will be to understand those who seek to destroy this process of love and freedom, to understand what motivates them toward hate and control, and to understand how to eliminate the seed of suffering. Deep in our DNA are the building blocks to allow the resolution of our intention to promote human life.

CHAPTER TEN

Now, Here, This

IT HAPPENS QUITE A BIT NOW. Not as often as I would like, of course, but so much more frequently than when I used to try so hard. I feel myself overcome with the present moment, and enter into it like into a skin. Writing this book has helped, because I am reminded of the present throughout the day. When the mornings are filled with writing and research, and thinking about how brain function facilitates a focus on current activity, the residue from these hours lingers into the evening, and serves as a frequent reminder to return to the present. The feeling of the effortless present comes along with this reminder almost every time, like a lonely boy and his dog.

In the years since I had my first experience of the golf club moving on its own, I have repeatedly seen the beneficial effect of letting the effortless present unfold in front of me. These experiences have led me to a very clear conclusion that, if a life involves paying full attention to this unfolding, it is enhanced immeasurably in all aspects. The relevance of this state of mind to our spiritual evolution remains an open scientific question, although I believe the unprovable notion that this process reflects the continued evolution of the human brain. Beyond these scientific and philosophical questions, however, I feel that the data are clear regarding the impact of the effortless present on daily life. Its benefit is certain.

I don't play golf so much anymore, though I love it when I play, and I miss it when I don't. I feel that golf gave me a glimpse of something I could have found anywhere, but that's probably wrong: I most likely needed golf to fully experience the effortless present. Other people would have needed something else, a karate class or a job in masonry. I had tried to experience oneness with the present in other endeavors, but was always left feeling stale and frustrated by my efforts. For me, golf on top of a landfill was the environment that allowed the richness of the moment to come to life. The pursuit of the effortless present in golf enabled me to delve so deeply into it that I could not forget it, and I have felt it since in every aspect of my life.

I remember feeling it strongly when I went to consult for the Duke football team for the first time. I was standing on the threshold of a major shift in my career, and I didn't want to make a mistake. I did not want to fail; I did not want to look down and get distracted by what I could lose. Yet going to football practice as a consultant sent me back to when I was a football player in college, and the ways I'd tried to invoke the effortless present on my own without having any idea of what I was doing.

When I was in college, I took a course entitled *The Varieties of Religious Experience*, based on the book of the same title by William James. We read about mystical experiences in the context of all the major religions. The professor, Malcolm Diamond, had written a book on the similarities and differences among Christianity, Judaism, Islam, Hinduism, and Buddhism, so we got a taste of everything. He was a warm and charismatic man in his mid fifties, and probably had more personal impact on me than any other Princeton professor. He always wore a tie and tweed jacket with actual patches on the elbows, and his hairline had receded significantly. At what appeared to be the vestige of a slight widow's peak, there were a few wild hairs sticking out in various directions; they reminded me of those Japanese soldiers from World War II who had been discovered in the 1950s, half-crazed and hiding out, still fighting a war on the front lines that had been surrendered behind them years ago.

My life at Princeton was saturated with failure. I had gone from being a self-assured class president and basketball captain at my high school to a struggling premed football player. For reasons still unknown to me, I was placed in the advanced chemistry and calculus classes as a freshman; after one test, the distribution of about 200 scores was placed on a bulletin board, with mine dead last. One of my fellow students had circled my outlying score and wrote next to it, "I am a moron."

I was able to keep my self-esteem afloat by becoming the starting wide receiver on the football team but, at Princeton, the response from my fellow students was more disdain than swoon. Professors also joined in the action, seeming to delight in the fact that we were a poor team even by Ivy League standards. Our losses seemed to solidify their view of the inverse correlation between intellectual ability and physical strength. I remember Nancy Cantor, now provost at Michigan University, being utterly astounded that, as a football player, I had gotten an *A* in her psychology course. (Ironically, Dr. Cantor has since conducted research on the values and behavior patterns of college athletes compared to other college students.) This derision was fairly universal and, as a result, the football team tended to cluster together like the members of any ethnic minority.

Malcolm Diamond was different from other professors. I met with him individually a few times when I'd missed class for away football games. He was not a football fan, but he had a genuine interest in my experience on the football field. He lectured a lot about Martin Buber's I-You experience, and how it connects people in a manner that transcends our existence as physical beings bound by time and lifts us toward God through each other. Being with Malcolm Diamond was a ripe environment for this type of experience, as his interests dwelled not on the reasons that you were meeting with him, but rather on the meeting itself. Each moment was new, and I could tell that he wasn't viewing me in the light of some kind of bias toward football players or mediocre students; he was just being with me. To a twenty-year-old growing accustomed to being treated with derision, his openness was quenching. One day during his lecture to the 200 or so students in his class, he discussed Buber's I-You experience from the perspective of complete attention on the current task, independent of selfish desire: "It's like a wide receiver in football," he said, "the emphasis is not on the *ego*, but on the *catch!*" I felt as if he were winking at me. His phrase resonated through me for years afterward: The focus should be on the experience of the moment, and not on the ego gratification and attention that will result from having completed the task.

That summer, just before my senior year, my closest friend, Steve Reynolds, and I obtained political internship positions in Washington, D.C. While living there in the sweaty swamp where the ancestors of our nation decided to locate our capital, I tried repeatedly to run wind sprints for the purpose of the experience, to work out in the sweltering heat with only the moment in mind. I failed convincingly. I was motivated by wanting to be great, wanting to see my name in headlines, wanting to earn stature among my peers, perhaps even to impress fellow students I did not know. But the actual moment of the catch left me flat, and I felt increasingly frustrated that I could not make myself practice for the purpose of the practice itself.

Steve and I lived together in the house of one of my sister's graduate school professors at American University, Margaret Rioch, in Bethesda, Maryland. As a testament to their superior intellect, Dr. Rioch and her husband had fled the heat of the area for the summer, and my sister had arranged for us to live in their house, free, while they were gone. (They must have snickered at us as veteran runners do at naïve marathon participants who are about to hit the twenty-mile wall for the first time.) Steve was the quarterback and captain of the football team, and we worked out together all summer in preparation for what was supposed to be the last season of our football careers. Steve traveled back to New Jersey some weekends, so I had large stretches of free time alone. I often wandered down to the library in their house, where there was an actual psychoanalyst's couch, hundreds of books on psychology and philosophy, and a section on mystical experience.

As I meandered through these texts, I was repeatedly exposed to the idea that focus on the current moment is bliss, yet I was never really able to attain it myself. I sat in front of the huge wheel that offered to change my life, and hoped and strained for it to turn, yet I had no idea how to make it turn. Each strenuous workout alienated me further from my enjoyment of football. I not only became frustrated at my inability to focus on the current moment, but I began to berate myself for failing at this endeavor, as though it were insubstantial merely to work all day at a shockingly boring job, then lift weights, run, and sprint pass patterns all evening. I was convinced that unless I performed these tasks for their own purpose, my quest was misguided and my goals were superficial and fruitless. The pressure became relentless, and I could not see that I was actually in the midst of a valuable and difficult exercise. My emphasis on succeeding at this task was too great; I did not understand at the time that this learning, like any other, is a process of stepping lightly and gradually toward the ideal. I had the childish notion that if I really were someone special, this new focus would come immediately and naturally to me. And since this view was so grandiose, I kept it to myself. Conveniently, it could never be challenged this way. So, at the time, I was never really able to learn how to develop my attention. I expected it to come to me and, if it didn't, I would berate myself for being ordinary, and try again and fail again. I was like the golfer who stubbornly prides himself on never having taken a lesson, yet never improves. I wanted to allow some kind of preordained ability to come to a full expression. If I could do that with no input from anyone else, it would sanctify my mission, and separate me from the rest of the struggling masses. I would never feel small again.

One of the problems with this immature strategy, however, was that since I didn't share my thoughts with anyone, I had no way to relax the intensity of my self-criticism. The failures led to shame and redoubled efforts to do it on my own. As in a convection oven, the energy I released was immediately funneled back within the system. I never talked with anyone about what I was doing until the day I walked out of football camp and didn't return my senior year. I told my close friends that I wasn't enjoying football camp, and they each looked at me quizzically, and asked, "Who *enjoys* football camp?"

I could afford to quit football—there were no athletic scholarships at Princeton, so my financial aid was not dependent upon my athletic participation. Perhaps if it had been so, I would have let myself to develop in the fits and starts characteristic of the rhythm of learning. I also might have given up altogether. For years, I dreamed that I was back at football camp, always at my actual age and level of physical conditioning and capacity to play (which at times was very slack). I guess a part of me knew that I had walked away from an opportunity to learn. Peculiarly, decades before I ever came to Duke, in the dream, the football jerseys were often not the orange-and-black colors of Princeton, but Duke blue and white.

Twenty years later, I had made it back to football camp but, this time, I was much more involved in what I was doing. I stood silently and watched. Sometimes, I had no idea what I was looking for but, since no one else knew what to expect from a performance-enhancement consultant, it was okay. The blue hue of the practice jerseys matched my dream exactly. The thought of fulfilling a decades' old unconscious destiny excited and embarrassed me. Was my failure to experience the effortless present as a player a long and meandering path to spending my life helping others achieve it? Or was I here merely because I had failed as a player, and longed to complete what was unfinished? I'm not sure that this mattered; I was here and I was present and nothing felt like it had to be changed.

When I played football as a wide receiver, I was usually concerned with my hands during games and practice—keeping them dry, warm, and, on game days, sticky, which was legal at the time. I developed a habit of keeping them protected inside my football pants which, unfortunately, carried over to the nonfootball hours of my day. As a receiver, I felt very dependent upon the health and welfare of my hands, and I could not simply turn off this dependence when I changed out of my football uniform. My protection of my hands continues to this day, perhaps as a vestige of their worth or, perhaps, in the hope that they'll be needed again. During practice at Duke that day, dressed in street clothes, I was having trouble finding a comfortable place for them. They weren't really necessary for my current activity. Putting them in my pockets seemed adolescent. Folding my arms across my chest felt too closed off and protective. Folding my hands together in front of me felt falsely pious and pretentious; putting them on my hips, too feminine. Twenty years ago, they had such purpose on the football field. The hands of youth have such grace and resilience; cuts would heal in a day or two. Now, cuts seem to linger for weeks before they disappear, calling out for the attention of their vigorous past.

I decided to let my hands go wherever they wanted to go. Like when I allowed the golf club to swing itself, I allowed my hands to find the position that was most comfortable for them. I disengaged from them. I shut down the connections between my frontal cortex and the hand area of my motor cortex, and allowed the hand movements to do their own little writhing dance. My attention shifted to the relevant present on the field, where our quarterback was being told that he was taking too many steps dropping back before his useful hands released a pass.

~

I WENT TO PLAY GOLF at the Duke course the other day. As I drove there, I recalled Harvey Penick's advice to drive unhurried to the course. I was never able to follow that advice. I was usually so excited to play that I always felt late, as though there wouldn't be enough time to get myself fully prepared before I played. I felt a need to be more than who I was, or at least to polish myself sufficiently to be in absolutely tip-top shape. When I arrived at the course, the hurrying would continue, and I would feel that I needed to get in more putting, more chipping, more tee balls. I would then feel a rush to get to the first tee, harboring a vague fear that the slowest foursome of the day was about to duck in front of my group. I would stand near the first tee like a rebounder prepared to box out any intruders.

Yet, this day, my drive was enriched by the present. It's possible that my goals for the day's round were not as intense as they once were, but this wouldn't completely account for the difference in my experience of getting to the course. The drive itself was full and absorbing, a striking contrast to the drives of years ago. I had covered this road hundreds of times yet, today, it stood out like a starkly illuminated corridor through a dull and dusky ether. The flagstones of a wall built alongside a driveway were radiant and stacked tenderly and naturally; someone had infused the project with an eye toward quality. I had noticed this wall so many times, but had never gleaned the attention that had been paid to craft: The builder cared not only about how the wall looked, but how it really was, and this was immediately evident that day. The beaver dam along the side of the road had become dangerously low, as it had not rained for weeks, and I wondered what beavers do in a drought. No work to do. What was the devil's playground for an idle beaver? Up ahead, the bends in the road seemed to carve the forest so delicately and minimally. Time was marching through this region, but technology's progress was being diverted, if only for a few decades.

As I arrived at the course that day, I felt a peace that was no longer unusual, yet was always pleasing. I was playing with my usual group, whom I hadn't seen for a while, and I looked forward to competing with them. Although my play was no longer as consistent as it was when I played more frequently, the good rounds were as good as before, and I had a feeling that today would be one of them. We went through the usual posturing and exaggerated shock at each other's handicaps, and settled upon the day's multiple wagers. I teed off relaxed, and glad to have come all this way from the New Jersey landfill.

As we walked down the first fairway, the banter turned to more substantial conversation or consideration of the upcoming shots. I drifted away from the group and approached my ball awaiting me. As I began to move into the consciousness of allowing the shot to manifest itself in front of me, I heard a gentle, almost perceptible voice coming from back in the dark tunnel of my psyche. It was a calm voice, almost recognizable, but slippery and hard to pinpoint. At first it sounded like a voice from a public address system on a navy ship. Then, it sounded like my father, or Professor Diamond, or even Roland Perlmutter. It was none of them and all of them. As I stood behind the ball and imagined the flight of the shot, mixed in with the descending murmur of other golfers and the wind and my own internal static, I distinctly heard the words, *Now . . . Hear . . . This*. At first, I interpreted the words as though they were being spoken by someone in the military, as though I were a soldier, and some-one was trying to get my attention. I awaited a further message, yet, the message was the same each time. *Now . . . Hear . . . This*. I finally realized that this *was* the message, and I had misinterpreted the middle word. It was not *hear*, but *here! "Now . . . Here . . . This."* It was the present bursting forth in song. I acquiesced to this voice of others coming from within; in each shot, I was still.

I don't think that I am capable of putting into words the richness of each shot that day. I did not have any mysterious experiences or a heavenly, sanctified hole-in-one, but I experienced the entire course as I walked through it. In a bunker, I felt all the grains of sand. On the green, I could feel the slope of every putt as though I had walked it a thousand times. Each shot seemed simple and unfathomable at the same time. My images of ball flight in my preshot routine were vivid and clear, including even a close-up perspective of where and how the ball would land. I had never before been more present, never more effortless. When we made the turn, my score was two or three shots lower than ever before. My partner and I were annihilating our opponents. I was having a wonderful time. It began to rain.

As the rain began to turn to a shower and my grips dampened, I felt a tenseness creep into my day. I wanted to continue the wonderful feeling of each shot exploding off my club face with power and grace. I loved the soft voice that was reminding me of the present moment before each shot. I also knew that I was going lower than I had ever gone before, and I wanted to finish with a number to symbolize the day. As I tried to hold on to these gifts, they began to slip away. My mood changed as abruptly as the weather. I wanted the outcome that had been promised me by the good fortune that I had been granted—no, that I had *earned*. I had entered into a state of focus and awareness because I had worked on it every day, and I felt that I deserved the riches I had bathed in moments ago. My swings became tense, and my images were fraught with fear of what could go wrong.

I began to long for what I didn't have: blue skies, dry ground, the feeling of the front nine. I became focused on wanting at least to continue trouncing my opponents, as if to vent my frustrations on them. At about the time my teeth began to grind, on the 11th tee, we heard the first rumblings of thunder. I denied it at first, insisting that it was a truck from the highway nearby. My partners knew that I was in the midst of a career round, and probably cast furtive glances at each other, but I was too focused to look at them. I had work to do now. Get out of my way. We headed on down the 11th fairway, and thunder rumbled again, this time unmistakable. "It's way far off," I said, continuing toward my ball, refusing to notice that they had all stopped in their tracks and were silently agreeing that they should not risk their lives any longer. As I headed up the side of the fairway toward the 11th green, out of the way of shots that would never come, one of them yelled to me that they were heading back.

In the seconds that it took for me to register this disheartening news, I was visited by a sudden image of what I remember about John F. Kennedy, Jr.'s death. I had read that the most likely end for him off the coast of Nantucket had been what is referred to as the *graveyard spin*. I had heard that John had been in a hurry that day. He had gone through his preflight checklist in the airport parking lot to save time, which had become precious to him. In the air over Nantucket, dusk had come earlier than he expected. The summer haze and the ocean and the gray-blue evening sky melded together, and all visual cues regarding his direction were lost. Inexperienced pilots like John lose their ability to fly in this situation, because the inner ear compensates for a slight turn, making them feel that they are flying straight and level when they are in fact slightly turning and descending. Without cues from the ground, they become completely confused. I could see John now, panicked but attempting to bear down on the task ahead of him, trying desperately to figure out where the horizon was, wondering whether he was going up or down, left or right. Should he trust his disoriented instincts or the baffling instrument panel in front of him? At some point during that spiral, John must have felt some regret over what he had done: not just that he had decided to go ahead and chance the flight, even though he knew it was dangerous, even though his wife's and sister-in-law's lives were in his hands. He must have also had some regret for who he was—no matter how much he had played it safe and reasonable compared to so many others in his extended family, the Kennedy drive was embedded in his DNA, and he was unable to stop himself from meeting an adventurous, early death.

What was this image telling me? Was I, like so many Kennedys, driving myself too hard toward an inherited vision for myself? Was I, too, unaware of my destination, spinning in space with engines blasting, going nowhere but down? I was willing to risk my life to finish this round. The circumstances seemed special, somehow. Anyone would continue, I thought. Yet today was no different than the rest of my life: There is no limit to what I would sacrifice to extend my reach. Goals are there to be vanquished. Achieve some more. Write the book. Do the research. More money. Bigger house. Improve the wife. Make the kids better than I could ever be.

As I turned to see my three partners slogging back up the 11th fairway toward the clubhouse, another image sprung into my mind. I had been playing basketball at a seven-foot hoop a few years ago with my two-year-old son. Each time I lifted him to the basket, he threw the ball down through the hoop with the vigor of a participant in an NBA slamdunk contest. I responded each time with my best Marv Albert "Yes!" causing him to burst into laughter with delight. There were no trophies handed out for this game, no bets paid on the 18th green, no scorecards to frame. There was only the moment and the connection and the graceful flow of our hands into the universe. As I walked back up the 11th fairway, I removed my soaked hat and breathed in the moist air while the sky lightly drummed fresh rain on my face. I had taken years to get here. Like a song that meanders away and away, then finally returns to G, I headed home.

I drove home slowly through the rain, again becoming absorbed in the details of the drive, the way life seemed to pucker in response to the rain, closing up and folding in, the feeling of uncertain contact between my tires and the puddles along the road. When I arrived home, I used the extra time I had to pay bills; by the time I was finished, the sun had come out and shone brightly on the wet, dripping world around our house.

I asked my four-year-old daughter to put the paid bills in the mailbox for the mailman to pick up. She was delighted at being given a meaningful task and anxiously agreed. I watched her from the upstairs window as she walked briskly toward the mailbox, driven not by a time schedule but by the transfer of her excitement into physical energy. Since placing the letters in the mailbox required her to set foot on the normally quiet street, and since she had learned the dangers of being in the street, she looked carefully up and down for cars. One was coming, and she stood stiffly facing the curbless street next to the mailbox, safely on the grass as though the natural laws of physics would not allow cars to tread there. She looked down the street again, and, quite unusually, another car was coming. She waited with resolute patience as the car passed. She continued to look down the street, and seemed to peer in one direction. I could not see the object of her stare; perhaps a car had stopped down the street. I later learned it was a distant orange construction barrel that she had mistaken for a fire. Upon realizing after a minute or two that the fire was neither diminishing nor growing, she slid her feet sideways under the mailbox so she could stay on the grass yet still have access to the mailbox door. With her feet pointing toward the street, she twisted around and curled her hand back above her head, opened the door, and slid the letters in. To my surprise, she raised the flag on the side of the mailbox to indicate that letters were contained within. As she skipped back inside, I gasped at the beauty of her enthusiasm, hoping to create a vacuum of the world from which this moment could never escape. I was older by a score, yet Professor Diamond's words still drifted by. I was finally able to focus on the catch.

~

MY FEVERISH DEVOTION to golf led me to understand the importance of so many other things in my life. I learned to be with myself, to trust myself, and to be with others in a way that had previously not been possible. Ultimately, I don't know if it was my neural circuitry, a spiritual force in the universe, or both, that led me down this path and allowed me access to these experiences of freedom and calm. But a door did open, and the moments of peace that I found on the other side of that door, I believe, are available to everyone.

It's natural to consider that only those who live in luxurious circumstances are candidates for these experiences, because everyone else is too busy trying to survive. Obviously, someone who is starving will have difficulty becoming absorbed in the current task if it doesn't involve satisfying her hunger. Everyone should have food, clothing, and shelter. Once they do, there are no excuses. Money does not buy this moment. It is available to everyone, whether on a golf course or a playground or a street corner.

Our brains have the capacity to make the decision to let the effortless present burst forth. Is this inspired by a spiritual force? I don't know. If there is a universal intelligence with a plan, how would it make itself known? In a Hollywood moment with hallelujah choruses and shafts of light? I doubt it. Such representations make the same point, but they're mere attention-grabbing icons of a slower-developing result. The miracles evident in today's world are numerous. Although in a snapshot it may not seem so, a look at humanity over the course of the last two millennia shows a slow progression from constant war toward peace, from poverty to wealth, from death to extended life. Terrorism has only been possible recently, as those without have learned what it might be like to have, and those who have are otherwise impenetrable. It will be a challenge to eliminate this behavior and the philosophy that inspires it. If we are to continue this progress toward heaven on earth, how will it look? Would we suddenly lose our innate tendencies to protect and fight and kill if necessary? Probably not. We will have to transform these basic instincts into acceptable skills. We will develop a society in which barbaric acts are eliminated, replaced by motoric acts that express the same energy and passion, yet do no harm. We will stop killing and engage in mastery. We romanticize swords transformed into ploughshares; while the current analogy may be that of M-16 rifles morphed into laptops, I think that hockey sticks and golf clubs are more likely. It is highly doubtful that the most efficient killing machine in the animal kingdom, the human, would ever lose the basic building blocks that have assured the survival of our genes through the course of evolution. Instead, their phenotypic expression into the world must be transformed into an acceptable, even palatable, form. Historians argue that this process began long ago, even before the ancient Olympics and Native American lacrosse games served to reduce the need for tribal warfare. If we are ever to reach a paradise in the future, this transformation would be complete. Soldiers become warriors in a mock battlefield of goal attainment. We would salute them with the vigor of conquering heroes because, in their peacetime achievements, our rapture with their form facilitates the process by which they are our protectors. If our enemy is similarly rapt, then we are safer than if we were standing behind the strongest military on earth.

Our absorption with the moment awakens us to the outside world. The effortless present of our stride along the earth connects us intimately with her surface. This connection is not theoretical but practical. Humans are physically connected with the external world as interdependent systems each bringing in and taking out. When we breathe, we bring in the cool air of the atmosphere and give out the carbon-dioxide–rich breath of life to the plants around us. The external world accepts our gift and replenishes. Everything we do, every feeling we have, interacts with the world, which responds to us, then crashes into us in the way that we have precipitated. Sometimes I feel like the world and I are a part of the same organism, and my breath is osmosis along the membrane line, giving, taking, flowing back and forth for the good of the whole that consumes us, all of us. My breath gives to the chlorophyll life around me, which fuels my neighbor with oxygen, regardless of how nosy she is. The process is so much bigger than our petty concerns, and it rides with us or without us. When we attend to the moment's interaction, we participate in this process. This engagement discourages suffering.

You cannot force a moment to be something that it's not. You cannot force yourself to be who you are not, but you can be who you are fully. A sand shot is not a curse; it is an opportunity. Buddhist philosophy teaches that enlightenment, Nirvana, is the same as Samsara, the daily cycle of life's little games. Nirvana is Samsara and Samsara is Nirvana. The story of the Buddhist monk is that he chops wood every day. When he reaches the pinnacle of spiritual experience, he still chops wood every day. Maybe these days he writes code in Java every day, but he does not change his activity when he attains Nirvana—yet his absorption into his moments writing code is complete. The bliss of our life is in its moments if we can allow them to be as they are. Respect for and devotion to this principle engorges life.

SELECTED REFERENCES

Barrow, G. W. S. *Kingship and Unity*. Toronto: University of Toronto Press, 1981.

Bechara, A., Damasio, H., Tranel, D., and Damasio, A. "Deciding advantageously before knowing the advantageous strategy." *Science*. 1997, 275, 1293–1295.

Boomer, Percy. *On Learning Golf*. New York: Alfred A. Knopf, 1946.

Buber, Martin. *I and Thou*. New York: Charles Scribner's Sons, 1970.

Casey, B. J., Giedd, J. N., and Thomas K. M. "Structural and functional brain development and its relation to cognitive development." *Biological Psychology*. 2000, 54: 241–257.

Carter, C. S., et al. "Anterior cingulate cortex, error detection, and the online monitoring of performance." *Science*, 1998, 280: 747–749.

Coop, Richard H., with Fields, Bill. *Mind Over Golf*. New York: Macmillan, 1993.

Csikszentmihalyi, Mihaly. *Flow: The Psychology of Optimal Experience*. New York: Harper and Row, 1990.

David-Neel, A. *Buddhism: Its Doctrines and Methods*. New York: St. Martin's Press, 1977.

Duncan, A. A. M. *Scotland: The Making of a Kingdom*. New York: Harper and Row, 1975.

Gallwey, Timothy W. *The Inner Game of Tennis* (revised edition). New York: Random House, 1997.

Gazzaniga, Michael S. *The New Cognitive Neurosciences*. England: Bradford Books, 1999.

Gould, E., et al. "Proliferation of granule cell precursors in the dentate gyrus of adult monkeys is diminished by stress." *Proceedings of the National Academy of Sciences*, 1998, 95 (March 16): 3168.

Gould, E., Reeves, A. J., Graziano, M. S., and Gross, C. G. 1999. "Neurogenesis in the neocortex of adult primates." *Science* (15 October), Vol. 286(5439): 548–552.

Haultain, Arnold. *The Mystery of Golf*. Bedford, MA: Applewood Books, 1965 (1908).

Herrigel, Eugen. *Zen In the Art of Archery*. New York: Random House, 1989.

Holmes, P. S., and Collins, D. J. "The PETTLEP approach to motor imagery: A functional equivalence model for sport psychologists." *Journal of Applied Sport Psychology*, 2001, 13 (1): 60–83.

Huang, Al, Chungliang, and Lynch, Jerry. *Thinking Body, Dancing Mind*. New York: Bantam Books, 1992.

Hyams, Joe. *Zen in the Martial Arts*. New York: Bantam Books, 1979.

Jackson, Susan A., and Csikszentmihalyi, Mihaly. *Flow in Sports*. Champaign, IL: Human Kinetics, 1999.

James, William. *The Principles of Psychology*. New York: Holt, Rinehart & Winston, 1890.

James William. *The Varieties of Religious Experience*. New York: Macmillan, 1961 (1902).

Jansma, J. M., Ramsey, N. F., Slagter, H. A., and Kahn, R. S. "Functional anatomical correlates of controlled and automatic processing." *Journal of Cognitive Neuroscience*, 2001, 13: 730–743.

Jha, A. and McCarthy, G. "The influence of memory load upon delay-interval activity in a working-memory task: an event-related functional MRI study. *Journal of Cognitive Neuroscience*, 2000 12: 90S–105S.

Kastner, S., et al. "Increased activity in human visual cortex during directed attention in the absence of visual stimulation." *Neuron*, 1999, 22: 751–761.

Lazar, S. W., Bush, G., Gollub, R. L., and Fricchione, G. L. "Functional brain mapping of the relaxation response and meditation." *Neuroreport*. 2000, 7: 1581–1585.

Lou, H. C., et al. "A ^{15}O-H$_2$O PET study of meditation and the resting state of normal consciousness." *Human Brain Mapping*, 1999, 7: 98–105.

Luria, A. R. *Higher Cortical Functions in Man*. New York: Basic Books, 1966.

Luria, A. R. *The Working Brain*. New York: Basic Books, 1973.

Mackenzie, Marlin M. with Denlinger, Ken. *Golf: The Mind Game*. New York: Dell, 1990.

McDonald, John. *Message of a Master*. California: New World Library, 1993.

Moran, Aidan P. *The Psychology of Concentration in Sport Performers*. East Sussex, UK: Psychology Press, 1996.

Murphy, Michael. *Golf in the Kingdom*. New York: Penguin Books, 1972.

Murphy, Michael, and White, Rhea A. *In the Zone*. New York: Penguin Books, 1995.

Newberg, A., et al. "The measurement of regional cerebral blood flow during the complex cognitive task of meditation: A preliminary SPECT study." *Psychiatry Research*, 2001, 106(2): 113–122.

Parrinder, G. *Mysticism in the World's Religions*. New York: Oxford University Press, 1976.

Passingham, Richard. *The Frontal Lobes and Voluntary Action*. Oxford University Press, 1993.

Penick, Harvey with Shrake, Bud. *Harvey Penick's Little Red Book*. New York: Simon & Schuster, 1992.

Posner, M. I., and Rothbart, M. K. "Attention, self-regulation, and consciousness." *Philosophical Transactions of the Royal Society, Biological Sciences,* 1998, 353: 1915–1927.

Ross, J. M. *Early Scottish History and Literature.* Glasgow: James Maclehose & Sons, 1884.

Ramnani, N., and Passingham, R. E. "Changes in the human brain during rhythm learning." *Journal of Cognitive Neuroscience,* 2001, 13: 952–966.

Rotella, Bob, with Cullen, Bob. *Golf Is not a Game of Perfect.* New York: Simon & Schuster, 1995.

Schneider, W., Pimm-Smith, M., and Worden, M. "Neurobiology of attention and automaticity." *Current Opinion in Neurobiology,* 1994, 4: 177–182.

Seligman, Martin. *Learned Optimism.* New York: Pocket Books, 1990.

Shoemaker, Fred, with Shoemaker, Pete. *Extraordinary Golf.* New York: G.P. Putnam's Sons, 1996.

Shulman, J. L., and Bowen, W. G. *The Game of Life.* Princeton University Press, 2001.

Sopa, G. L., and Hopkins, J. *Practice and Theory of Tibetan Buddhism.* New York: Grove Press, 1976.

Stace, W. T. *Mysticism and Philosophy.* New York: Macmillan, 1960.

Tendzin, Ösel. *Buddha In the Palm of Your Hand.* Boulder, CO: Shambala Press, 1982.

Trungpa, Chogyam. *The Myth of Freedom.* Boulder, CO: Shambala Press, 1976.

ACKNOWLEDGMENTS

IT HAS TAKEN ME SEVERAL YEARS to complete this book, and there are many people who have made important contributions to its development along the way. Since the themes are very personal, a complete acknowledgment would include most of the people I have known. I am sure to have forgotten key people; let me apologize to them in advance.

My editor, Jeff Neuman, and my agent, Faith Hamlin, have been invaluable at every stage. The two of them encouraged me to shift the focus of the book to what I really thought and felt about the golf experiences I had actually had, and to write about the science behind them. They have been essential guides through this transformation, and pushed me to do things I never would have been able to do alone.

Dick Coop has been as good a mentor as anyone could hope for. He taught me about sport psychology and introduced me to the professional golf world with no other motive than to pass on the wealth of information and understanding contained in his huge heart.

Although the final responsibility of the accuracy of the science, history, and religion discussed in the book are with me, several people read sections of the book to offer their advice, and added needed encouragement along the way. Dan Kenna, Terry Goldberg, Robert Bilder, Joel Kleinman, Dave Pickar, and John Gilmore were particularly helpful. Danny Weinberger's advice was also helpful, and his interest in the book and his unbridled enthusiasm for the topic was inspiring. Doug Tibbetts gave sage advice as well, especially in the early stages of deciding what direction the book should take. George Gopen's excitement about writing echoed through each page.

Roland Perlmutter is a composite character based upon a number of people I have either known, interviewed, or whose work I have studied. The science he describes is as true as I can communicate it. My editor and I felt that people would understand the science better if it were described in the context of the enthusiasm that many of my colleagues and I feel about it.

Many people have encouraged me to write this book; all of it was needed. In particular, Jeff Foote, Xavier Amador, Jim Garofalou, Jamie Mead, and John Strauss impressed upon me to work from inside to out. My chairman, Ranga Krishnan, deserves special mention because every minute I worked on this book was a minute that I did not work on my research in his department, yet he encouraged me anyway. Susan Arellano got me to see that the truth is much more interesting than fiction, and helped point me in that direction.

Leigh Coughenour, Susan Shortel, Karen Emberger, and Meg Poe completed factfinding and literature searches. Chuck Eesley worked on the brain figure and helped with the reference list. Cyndie Gregory had a crucial role in my interactions with the outside world about the book.

There are several people who provided me with important opportunities that allowed the circumstances for me to write, especially Chris Kennedy, Charlie Rozanski, Richard Surwit, Herb Sendek, Alan Breier, Hap Zarzour, Jackie Silar, Jan Ogilvie, Richard Sykes, Greg McCarthy, Joe McEvoy, and Ken Davis. Jeffrey Lieberman has generated several careers worth of opportunities for me.

Phil Harvey has been a tremendously generous friend and colleague.

Ed Ibarguen has not only been personally helpful with his support and insights about golf, but he and his staff have provided me with rich opportunities for my sport psychology work to thrive.

I have learned a lot from my regular golf partners over the years, especially Bob Stanger; Larry Eimers; Lex Alexander; Steve Herman; Jim Gray; Dave Van Voorhees; Eric Ardery; my father, Jack Keefe; Austin David; Dave Hollander; Victoria Morgan; and Doug Tibbetts.

A lot of this book has a personal touch, and I hope that I have represented fairly those who have touched me and shaped the way I feel about the world. My father, mother, brother, and sister gave me much more than what was required by their job descriptions, and their love provided an environment for thriving.

This book is dedicated to my wife Caren and our children. Caren willingly gave up years of our evenings and mornings together and trudged through countless chores alone while I worked on this book. Our children had less choice, but sacrificed just the same. It was a genuine group effort. Without your help, I may have finished the book, but it would never have been complete.

INDEX

ABOUT THE AUTHOR

DR. RICHARD KEEFE is a clinical psychologist, neuroscience researcher, and Director of Sport Psychology at Duke University. Dr. Keefe has published more than seventy-five articles and three books on brain disorders, primarily schizophrenia. His current research uses functional Magnetic Resonance Imaging (fMRI) to investigate how the brain initiates and experiences complex actions. He consults to numerous college and professional athletes, coaches, and teams, including those from Duke, North Carolina State, the NBA, MLB, NFL, and NHL. He works with golfers at all levels and has helped individuals prepare for everything from high-school tournaments to the Masters. He graduated in 1980 from Princeton University, where he was a starting wide receiver on the football team. His research there focused on religious and nonreligious mystical experience.

Printed in the United States
By Bookmasters